Practical Procedures in the Emergency Department

John Bache FRCS, FFAEM
Consultant in Accident and Emergency Medicine
Leighton Hospital, Crewe, Cheshire, England

Carolyn Armitt RGN, TNCC(P)
Sister and Emergency Nurse Practitioner
Accident and Emergency Department,
Leighton Hospital, Crewe, Cheshire, England

Cathy Gadd RGN, TNCC(P), APLS(I)
Sister and Emergency Nurse Practitioner
Accident and Emergency Department,
Leighton Hospital, Crewe, Cheshire, England

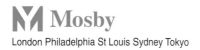

Mosby

London Philadelphia St Louis Sydney Tokyo

Publisher	**Jill Northcott**
Development Editor	**Gillian Harris**
Project Manager	**Louise Patchett**
Design	**Greg Smith**
Layout	**Rob Curran**
Cover Design	**Greg Smith**
Production	**Hamish Adamson**
Index	**Nina Boyd**

Copyright © 1998 Mosby International Limited

Published by Mosby, an imprint of Mosby International Limited, Lynton House, 7–12 Tavistock Square, London WC1H 9LB, UK

ISBN 0 7234 3013 6

Printed by Grafos S.A. Arte sobre papel, Barcelona, Spain

For full details of all Mosby titles, please write to Mosby International Publishers Limited, Lynton House, 7–12 Tavistock Square, London WC1H 9LB, UK.

A CIP catalogue record for this book is available from the British Library.

Library of Congress Cataloging-in-Publication Data has been applied for.

Contents

MISCELLANEOUS PROCEDURES

Introduction

The predecessor of this book, *A Colour Atlas of Nursing Procedures in Accidents and Emergencies*, was first published in 1985. Although some procedures remain unchanged, obviously new techniques have been established and new equipment has been introduced. More fundamental, however, is a change in the underlying ethos of emergency medicine. As in other branches of medicine, boundaries have become less distinct, so that many procedures which were once confined to one particular group of staff may now be undertaken by doctors, nurses, or paramedics. The vast clinical experience of senior nurses in the emergency department has been increasingly recognized in the expanding role of the emergency nurse practitioner.

Emergency medicine is an intensely practical specialty, and this is an intensely practical book. It provides a step-by-step approach to a wide range of practical procedures, and each procedure described is complete in itself. The book is intended to be the clinical equivalent of an illustrated book of recipes: for each procedure we have described the uses, the equipment required, and the practical aspects of the procedure. We hope that the book does not lie unused on the shelf, but that it is consulted on a daily basis by emergency nurse practitioners, senior and junior nurses, and doctors of all grades. We anticipate that it is also useful for general practitioners, nurses in the community, and paramedics. The procedures described range from those undertaken many times each day in every emergency department to those required only rarely. We have not included procedures which we feel will probably be familiar to every nurse.

It should be noted that when describing the equipment required for plasters of Paris etc, we have given the sizes for an average adult. Obviously these may need to be adjusted for specific patients.

While writing this book, we have received assistance from families, friends, and colleagues. We would particularly like to thank Steve Neilson for the photographic work. We are also grateful to Peter Dowds for helping with parts of the text, and to Roy and Jean Burton for typing the first draft. We have received encouragement from all the staff in the Emergency Department at Leighton Hospital. We are grateful to Adam Armitt and to those patients and colleagues who have agreed to allow us to photograph them. We would like to thank Nicola Horton, who provided enormous and friendly support when we were in difficulties. Finally, the book would not have been possible without the support of Lorraine, Sarah, Pauline, Joseph and David.

John Bache
Carolyn Armitt
Cathy Gadd

This book is dedicated to the memory of

Jill Dodds

1962–1996

A truly inspirational and courageous young lady

Soft cervical collar

USES
- Injuries of the cervical spine, including whiplash injuries.
- Torticollis.
- Cervical spondylosis.

EQUIPMENT
- Cervical collar of suitable size; various types are available.

PROCEDURE
1. Expose the neck.
2. Remove any jewellery that might be obstructive, e.g. necklaces.
3. Position the shaped area of the collar under the chin while the patient is looking straight ahead.
4. Fasten the collar into position, ensuring that it fits firmly but comfortably (Figures 1A and 1B).

Figure 1A

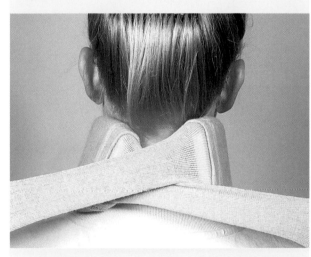

Figure 1B

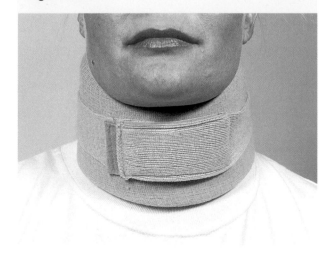

Advice to patients with whiplash injuries

- Do not wear the collar all the time, i.e. remove it regularly to avoid becoming reliant upon it.
- Repeat the following exercises ten times each, four times daily:
  a) Using smooth slow movements, draw yourself up straight, tuck in your chin to make a double chin, then relax.
  b) Turn your head round to look over each shoulder.
  c) Look straight ahead and try to touch your shoulder with your ear.
  d) Bend your neck forwards and backwards.
- The following may also help:
  a) Apply an ice pack to the painful side for 10 minutes, four times daily.
  b) If an ice pack is too uncomfortable, use a hot water bottle for 15 to 20 minutes.
- The collar should usually be worn at night. Use one or two pillows so that the head can be kept straight, in line with the back.

This advice may change for torticollis and cervical spondylosis. Follow the specific advice you are given.

Hard cervical collar

USE
- To immobilize the cervical spine following trauma.

EQUIPMENT
- Two-piece hard cervical collar.
- Two sandbags or purpose-made foam head blocks.
- Elastic adhesive tape, 7.5 cm wide.
- Scissors.
- Suction.

PROCEDURE
Two people are required for this procedure. Suction should be available in case the patient vomits.
1. Throughout the procedure, one person immobilizes the cervical spine, explaining to the patient the importance of not moving the neck.
2. Select the correct size of collar, following the manufacturer's instructions.
3. The second person performs the remainder of the procedure.
4. Remove all jewellery from the patient's neck.
5. Position the front piece of the collar beneath the patient's chin, wrapping the retaining strap around the back of the neck and fastening it firmly at the front (Figure 2A).
6. Slide the back piece centrally behind the patient's head, bringing both straps around to attach to the front piece. The collar should now be holding the neck securely (Figure 2B). Place sandbags on either side of the patient's neck to prevent any lateral movement.
7. To complete the procedure, secure a length of elastic adhesive tape across the forehead, anchoring it firmly to the sides of the trolley or spinal board, in order to ensure immobilization of the neck. Alternatively, purpose-made foam head blocks can be used (Figure 2C).

Figure 2A

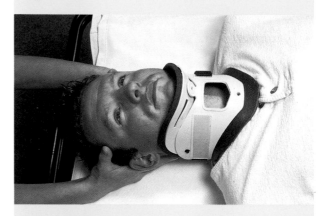

Figure 2B

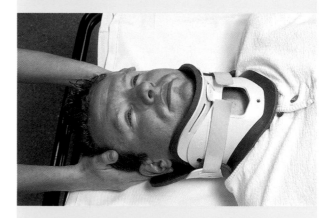

Figure 2C

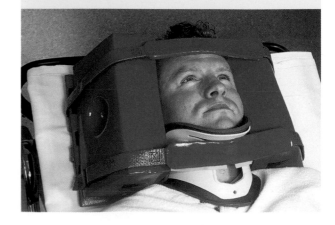

Elasticated tubular support to the elbow

USES
- Joint effusions and sprains.
- Soft tissue injuries.
- After aspiration of the joint or a bursa.
- After removal of a plaster of Paris.

EQUIPMENT
- Elasticated tubular support, 8.5 cm wide.
- Scissors.

PROCEDURE
1. Make sure the patient is comfortable, and expose the arm.
2. Cut a length of about 30 cm of elasticated tubular support.
3. Place the elasticated tubular support around the elbow, from one handspan above to one handspan below (Figure 3).
4. If additional support is required, apply a double layer of elasticated tubular support but leave a 2 cm gap between the two layers to prevent a tourniquet-type effect.
5. Check the radial pulse to ensure the circulation is satisfactory.

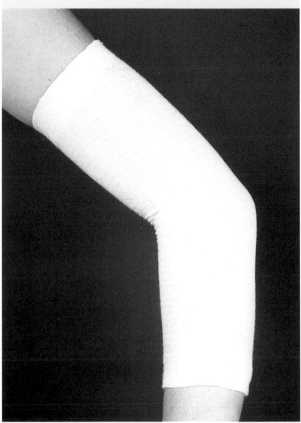

Figure 3

Advice to patients

- Keep the support clean and dry.
- Remove the support when washing the arm, then re-apply; the support can be washed separately.
- Keep the support smooth and remove it at night to prevent constriction.
- Exercise and/or elevate the arm as advised.
- Apply an ice pack to the swollen area for 10 minutes, up to four times daily.
- Use the support for as long as required.

Elasticated tubular support to the wrist

USES
- Joint effusions and sprains.
- Soft tissue injuries.
- After aspiration of a ganglion.
- After removal of a plaster of Paris.

EQUIPMENT
- Elasticated tubular support, 7 cm wide.
- Scissors.

PROCEDURE
1. Make sure the patient is comfortable, and expose the arm.
2. Cut a length of about 35 cm of elasticated tubular support.
3. Cut a small hole about 6 cm from one end for the thumb.
4. Slide the elasticated tubular support along the patient's forearm, with the thumb through the hole, leaving the elbow and knuckles exposed (Figures 4A and 4B).
5. If additional support is required, apply a double layer of elasticated tubular support, snipping the small hole about 6 cm from the folded edge. Leave a 2 cm gap between the two layers at the upper end, to prevent a tourniquet-type effect.
6. Check the colour and warmth of the hand to ensure that the circulation is satisfactory.

Advice to patients

- Keep the support clean and dry.
- Remove the support when washing the arm, then re-apply; the support can be washed separately.
- Keep the support smooth and remove it at night in order to prevent constriction.
- Exercise and/or elevate the arm as advised.
- Apply an ice pack to the swollen area for 10 minutes, up to four times daily.
- Use the support for as long as required.

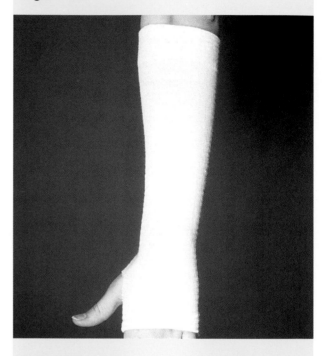

Figure 4A

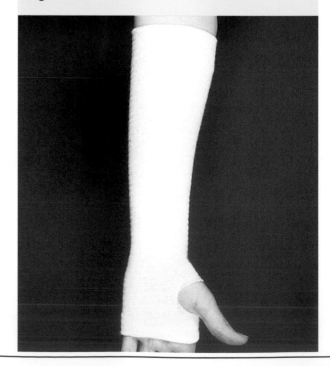

Figure 4B

5.

Crepe bandage to the elbow

USES
- Support for sprains or bruises.
- As a pressure dressing, to reduce swelling or prevent bleeding.
- After removal of a plaster of Paris.

EQUIPMENT
- Crepe bandage, 10 cm wide.
- Elastic adhesive tape, 2.5 cm wide.
- Scissors.

PROCEDURE
1. Make sure the patient is comfortable, and expose the arm.
2. With the elbow slightly flexed, apply the crepe bandage in a spiral fashion, from one handspan below the elbow to one handspan above the elbow.
3. Secure with elastic adhesive tape (Figure 5).

Advice to patients

- Keep the bandage clean and dry.
- Remove the bandage when washing the arm, then re-apply.
- Exercise and/or elevate the arm as advised.
- Use the bandage for as long as required.

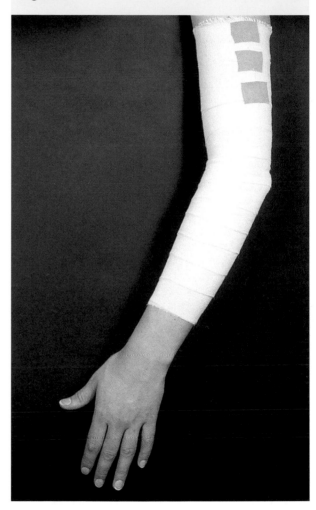

Figure 5

Crepe bandage to the wrist

USES
- Support for sprains or bruises.
- As a pressure dressing, to reduce swelling or prevent bleeding.
- After removal of a plaster of Paris.

EQUIPMENT
- Crepe bandage, 7.5 cm wide.
- Elastic adhesive tape, 2.5 cm wide.
- Scissors.

PROCEDURE
1. Make sure the patient is comfortable, expose the arm, and request that the hand is placed in a neutral position.
2. Anchor the crepe bandage around the wrist with a fixing turn.
3. Proceed around the hand in a figure-of-eight fashion, at least twice (Figures 6A and 6B).
4. Continue up the forearm in a spiral fashion, covering two-thirds of the width of the crepe bandage with each turn, to about 3 cm below the elbow.
5. Secure with elastic adhesive tape.
6. Ensure that the fingers and thumb are exposed so that they can be exercised (Figure 6C).

Advice to patients

- Keep the bandage clean and dry.
- Remove the bandage when washing the arm, then re-apply.
- Exercise and/or elevate the arm as advised.
- Use the bandage for as long as required.

Figure 6A

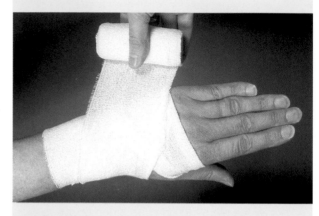

Figure 6B

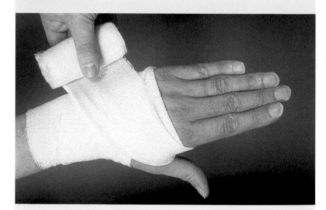

Figure 6C

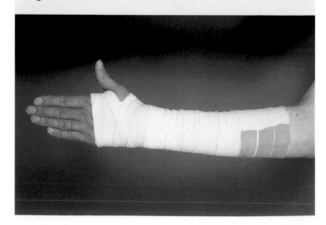

7.

Wrist brace

USES
- Tenosynovitis of the wrist.
- Certain soft tissue injuries and inflammatory conditions of the wrist.
- After removal of a plaster of Paris.

EQUIPMENT
- Wrist brace of appropriate size, with or without a thumb extension. Wrist braces are usually sized small, medium, or large and are marked for use on the left or the right wrist.

PROCEDURE
1. Make sure the patient is comfortable, expose the arm, and request that the wrist is placed in a neutral position.
2. Position the wrist brace with the metal strip running along the palmar aspect of the wrist.
3. Anchor the velcro straps across the wrist and between the thumb and index finger, ensuring that the wrist brace fits snugly around the wrist and hand but permits full movement of the fingers—and of the thumb if a thumb extension is not used (Figure 7).

Figure 7

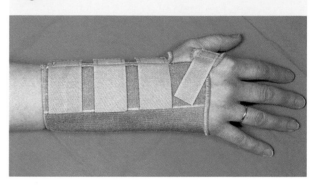

Advice to patients

- Keep the brace clean and dry; it may be removed to enable the patient to wash.
- Exercise the arm as advised.
- Wear the brace for as long as advised.

Thumb spica

USES
- Fractures, sprains, or bruises of the thumb.
- Following reduction of a dislocated thumb.

EQUIPMENT
- Cotton tubular bandage, 1.5 cm wide.
- Elastic adhesive tape, 2.5 cm wide.
- Scissors.
- A crepe bandage, 5 cm wide, for a patient who is allergic to elastic adhesive tape.

PROCEDURE
1. Ensure that the patient is not allergic to elastic adhesive tape—if the patient is, see the procedure using crepe bandage (below).
2. Cut a length of about 10 cm of cotton tubular bandage. Slide it over the thumb and fold back the cut edges, leaving the tip of the thumb exposed.
3. Cut about eight pieces of elastic adhesive tape of varying lengths from 8 cm to 15 cm.
4. Apply the lengths of elastic adhesive tape from the tip of the thumb to the base, overlapping each piece slightly and forming a 'V' from the nail to the base of the first metacarpal. Snip the tape as required (Figures 8A and 8B) around the web space of the hand. Take care not to apply the elastic adhesive tape under tension, because this may restrict the circulation.
5. Complete the spica by applying a length of elastic adhesive tape around the wrist to anchor the ends of the tape: leave a 2 cm gap in order to avoid constriction (Figure 8C).
6. To ensure that the circulation is satisfactory, press the thumb tip and check that the normal colour returns immediately.

USING CREPE BANDAGE
Crepe bandage should be used in patients who are allergic to elastic adhesive tape:
1. Secure the crepe bandage around the wrist with two turns.
2. Moving up the thumb, wind the crepe bandage around and back to the hand in a figure-of-eight fashion until complete (Figure 8D). The spica should feel firm and supportive but not too tight.
3. Secure the end of the crepe bandage with two pieces of elastic adhesive tape, which must not be in contact with the patient's skin (Figure 8E).
4. To ensure that the circulation is satisfactory, press the thumb tip and check that the normal colour returns immediately.

Figure 8A

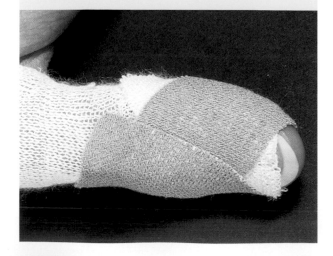

Figure 8B

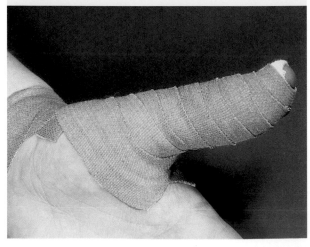

Figure 8C

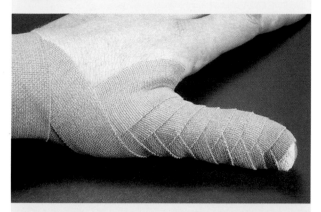

Figure 8D

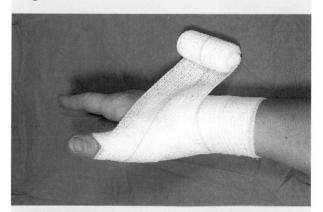

Figure 8E

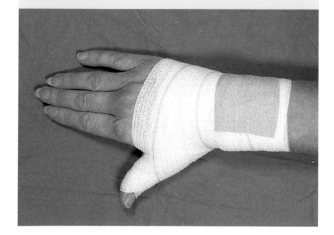

Advice to patients

- Keep the thumb spica clean and dry.
- Elevate the hand as much as possible. Wear a high sling (if provided with one) for as long as instructed (Procedure 12).
- If the thumb becomes discoloured (other than with delayed bruising) or numb, or severe pain or tingling develop, seek further medical attention.
- Exercise the arm as advised.
- Wear the thumb spica for as long as advised.

Neighbour ('buddy') strapping

USES
- Fractures, sprains, or bruises of the fingers or toes.
- After reduction of fractured or dislocated fingers or toes.

EQUIPMENT
- Cotton tubular bandage, 1.5 cm wide.
- Elastic adhesive tape, 2.5 cm wide.
- Scissors.

PROCEDURE
1. Make sure the patient is comfortable, and expose the injured fingers or toes.
2. Cut two lengths of cotton tubular bandage, each about 12 cm in length.
3. Slide the cotton tubular bandage onto the two selected digits and turn over the cut edges in order to prevent fraying.
4. Cut two lengths of elastic adhesive tape and apply one above and the other below the proximal interphalangeal joint, strapping the two digits together (Figures 9A and 9B).
5. Ensure that the strapping is comfortable. A high sling may be required in order to elevate the hand (Procedure 12).

Figure 9A

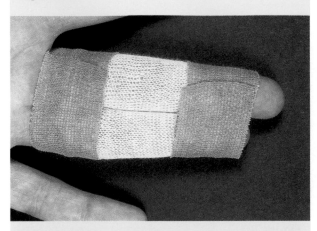

Figure 9B

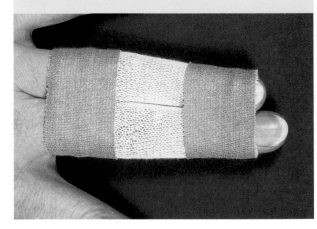

Advice to patients

- Keep the neighbour strapping clean and dry.
- Exercise the fingers or toes within the neighbour strapping.
- Wear the neighbour strapping for as long as advised.

Mallet splint

USE
- Mallet finger—due to rupture of the terminal extensor tendon or avulsion of a fragment of its bony insertion.

EQUIPMENT
- Mallet finger splint of the correct size; various types are available.
- Adhesive felt, 5 mm thick.
- Elastic adhesive tape, 2.5 cm wide.
- Scissors.
- Non-allergenic tape, for a patient who is allergic to elastic adhesive tape.

PROCEDURE
1. Ensure that the patient is not allergic to elastic adhesive tape—if the patient is, substitute with a non-allergenic tape.
2. Expose the injured finger and remove any rings. Wash and dry the finger (Figure 10A).
3. Slide the mallet finger splint onto the finger, ensuring that the terminal joint (the distal interphalangeal joint) is straight and neither flexed nor hyperextended. To achieve this, the end of the splint can be padded with a small piece of adhesive felt (Figures 10B and 10C). Ensure that the proximal interphalangeal joint is not splinted. The finger should fit comfortably but firmly within the splint.
4. Attach the splint to the finger with elastic adhesive tape (Figure 10D).

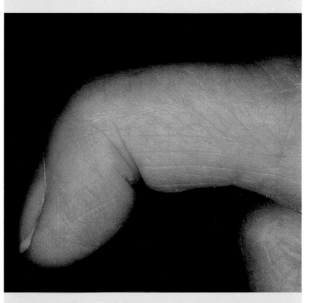

Figure 10A

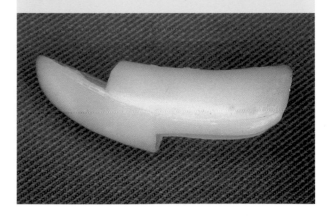

Figure 10B

Figure 10C

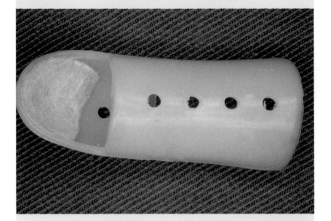

Figure 10D

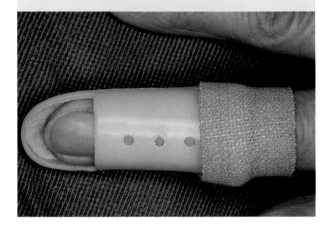

Advice to patients

- The injury usually takes about six weeks to heal, and the splint must not be removed during this period. If it is removed, even very briefly, the injured tendon or bone is likely to separate again.
- Keep the finger as clean and dry as possible; a finger stall may be useful.
- If the finger becomes discoloured (other than with delayed bruising) or numb, or severe pain or tingling develop, seek further medical attention.
- Exercise the other joints of the hand, including the proximal interphalangeal joint of the injured finger.

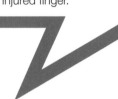

Broad arm (triangular) sling

USES
- Fractures of the clavicle, scapula, humerus, elbow, forearm, wrist, or metacarpals.
- After reduction of a dislocated shoulder, dislocated elbow, or dislocated fingers or thumb.
- Infections of the arm, including olecranon bursitis.
- To support an above-elbow plaster of Paris cast, or an injured arm.

EQUIPMENT
- Sling.
- Safety pin (for an adult).
- Elastic adhesive tape, 2.5 cm wide (for a child).
- Scissors.

PROCEDURE
1. Undress the patient down to the waist if the sling is to be worn under the clothes. Remove all jewellery from the neck and from the injured arm.
2. Make sure the patient is comfortable, and place the elbow at a right angle.
3. Place the long straight side of the sling parallel to the sternum and place the apex of the sling behind the injured arm. Extend the upper end of the sling over the opposite shoulder (Figure 11A).
4. Bring the lower end of the sling over the shoulder of the injured arm. Tie the two ends behind the neck.
5. Secure the elbow in the sling using a safety pin for an adult or elastic adhesive tape for a child (Figure 11B).

Advice to patients
- Exercise the uninjured joints of the arm.
- If the sling is to be removed at night, a relative should be shown how to re-apply it.
- The sling should be worn for as long as advised.

Figure 11A

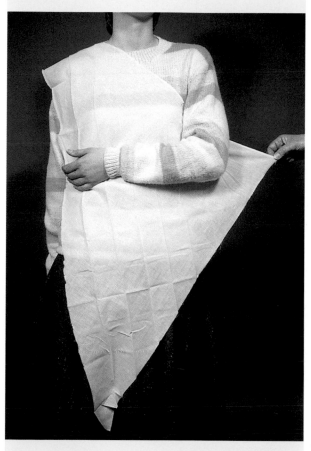

Figure 11B

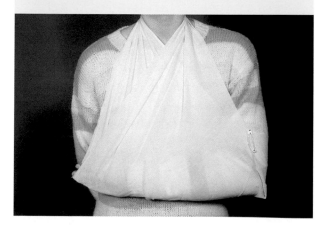

High sling

USES
- As for a broad arm (triangular) sling.
- To stop haemorrhage (together with a pressure dressing).
- To reduce swelling of the forearm, wrist, or hand.
- To provide elevation of a child's arm, without using a safety pin (Method B).

EQUIPMENT
Method A
- Sling.
- Two safety pins (for an adult).
- One self-locking safety pin (for a child).
- Elastic adhesive tape, 2.5 cm wide (for a child).
- Scissors.

Method B
- Sling.

PROCEDURE
Method A
1. Undress the patient down to the waist if the sling is to be worn under the clothes. Remove all jewellery from the neck and from the injured arm.
2. Make sure the patient is comfortable.
3. Place the long straight side of the sling parallel to the sternum and place the apex of the sling behind the injured arm. Extend the upper end of the sling over the opposite shoulder (Figure 12A).
4. Bring the lower end of the sling over the shoulder of the injured arm. Tie the two ends behind the neck.
5. Secure the elbow in the sling with a safety pin for an adult or elastic adhesive tape for a child (Figure 12B).
6. Raise the hand of the injured arm up to the opposite shoulder and secure the sling with a safety pin (self-locking type for a child) (Figure 12C).

Method B
1. Undress the patient down to the waist if the sling is to be worn under the clothes. Remove all jewellery from the neck and from the injured arm.
2. Make sure the patient is comfortable.
3. Tuck the right-angled corner of the sling under the axilla of the injured arm (Figure 12D).

4. Place the injured arm over the sling, requesting the patient to bend the elbow and reach upwards towards the opposite shoulder.
5. Bring the lower end of the sling up and around the elbow to the patient's back.
6. The two ends of the sling should now meet approximately between the patient's shoulder blades, where they can be tied in a knot (Figure 12E).
7. Tuck the remaining loose end under the elbow of the injured arm (Figure 12F).

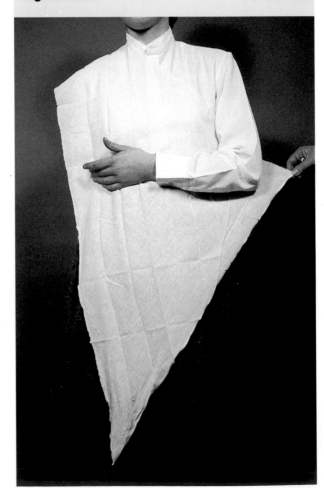

Figure 12A

Figure 12B

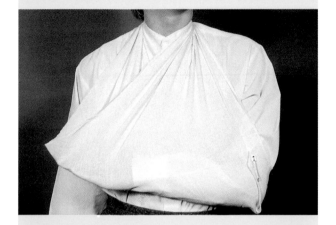

Figure 12C

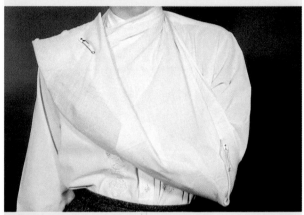

Figure 12D

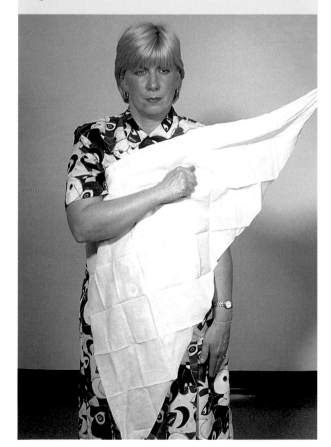

Figure 12E

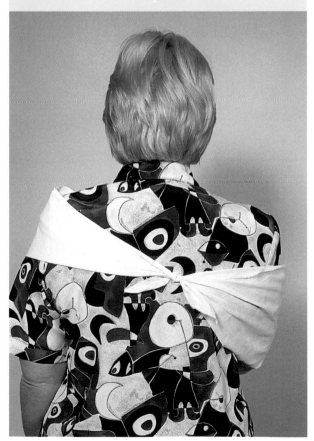

Figure 12F

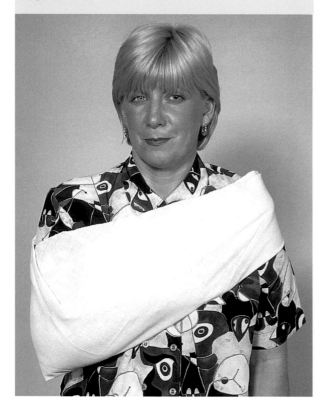

Advice to patients

- Exercise the uninjured joints of the arm.
- Remove the sling at night but try to sleep with the injured arm resting up on two pillows. A relative should be shown how to re-apply the sling.
- The sling should be worn for as long as advised.

Collar-and-cuff

USES
- Fracture of the neck of the humerus.
- To support an above-elbow plaster of Paris cast, or a U-slab plaster.

EQUIPMENT
- Collar-and-cuff; various types are available.
- Tie fastener.
- Elastic adhesive tape, 2.5 cm wide.
- Scissors.

PROCEDURE
1. The collar-and-cuff may be worn under the clothes or over the clothes, depending upon the nature of the injury and how much mobility is to be encouraged.
2. If it is to be worn under the clothes, undress the patient down to the waist and remove all jewellery from the neck and from the injured arm. Wash and dry the axilla.
3. Position the injured arm with the elbow at a right angle or higher.
4. Cut about 120 cm length of collar-and-cuff and encircle it in a figure-of-eight around the neck and around the wrist of the injured arm.
5. Secure with a tie fastener (Figure 13A), snipping off the surplus sharp end of the tie fastener.
6. Cover the tie fastener with elastic adhesive tape to ensure a smooth, secure finish (Figure 13B).
7. To ensure that the circulation is satisfactory, check the radial pulse and the colour and sensation of the fingers.
8. If an inescapable collar-and-cuff is required (e.g. for children), it is advisable to continue the elastic adhesive tape from the wrist to the neck.
9. If the collar-and-cuff is to be worn over the clothes, ensure that the patient can slip it over the head and wrist.

Advice to patients

- Exercise the uninjured joints of the arm.
- If the arm becomes discoloured (other than with delayed bruising) or numb, seek further medical attention.
- Wear the collar-and-cuff during the day and at night if it is applied under the clothes—if it is applied over the clothes, wear as instructed.
- The collar-and-cuff should be worn for as long as advised.
- To prevent the arm from rubbing against the chest, a tee-shirt or a vest, split at the shoulder, may be worn.

Figure 13A

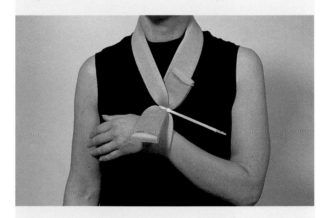

Figure 13B

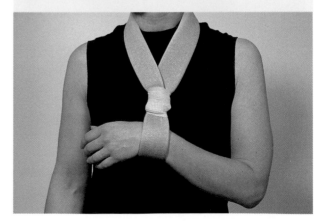

Elasticated tubular support to the knee

USES
- Joint effusions and sprains.
- Soft tissue injuries.
- After aspiration of the knee joint or a bursa.
- After removal of a plaster of Paris.

EQUIPMENT
- Elasticated tubular support, 9.5 cm wide.
- Applicator.
- Scissors.

PROCEDURE
1. Make sure the patient is comfortable, and expose the leg.
2. Cut a length of about 35 cm of elasticated tubular support.
3. Thread the support onto the applicator.
4. Pass the applicator over the knee and position it a handspan above the knee.
5. Remove the upper end of the elasticated tubular support from the applicator and position it around the thigh (Figure 14A).
6. Covering the knee with the elasticated tubular support, slowly remove the applicator towards the foot, finishing a handspan below the knee (Figure 14B).
7. If additional support is required, apply a double layer of elasticated tubular support but leave a 2 cm gap between the two layers to prevent a tourniquet-type effect.
8. Ensure that the circulation is satisfactory by checking the colour and warmth of the foot.

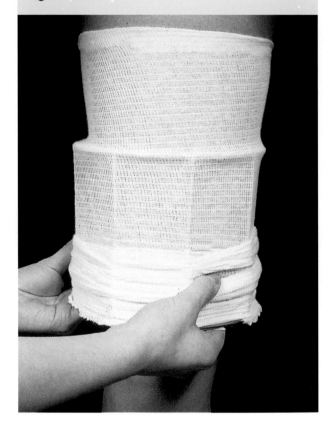

Figure 14A

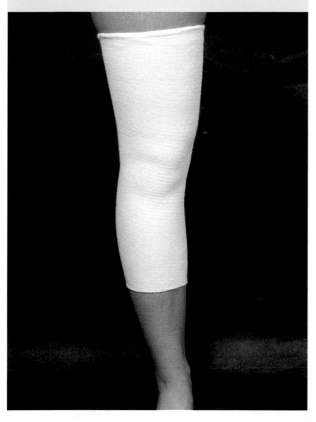

Figure 14B

Advice to patients

- Keep the support clean and dry.
- Remove the support when washing the leg, then re-apply; the support can be washed separately.
- Keep the support smooth and remove it at night in order to prevent constriction.
- Follow the **NICER** regimen for acute injuries:

  N: **Non-steroidal anti-inflammatory agents** may be of benefit;

  I: Apply an **Ice** pack to the swollen area for 10 minutes, up to four times daily, and remove the elasticated tubular support before applying the ice pack;

  C: Use the elasticated tubular support for **Compression** and for support for as long as required;

  E: **Elevate** the limb higher than the level of the waist while sitting or lying;

  R: **Rest** or exercise the leg as advised. Exercise the quadriceps musculature by holding the foot at a right angle and tightening the muscle at the front of the thigh; raise the straightened leg for five seconds, then lower it slowly; rotate the ankle clockwise and anti-clockwise. Repeat these exercises for five minutes every hour during the day.
- A walking aid may be provided (Procedure 26).

Elasticated tubular support to the ankle

USES
- Joint effusions and sprains.
- Soft tissue injuries.
- After removal of a plaster of Paris.

EQUIPMENT
- Elasticated tubular support, 8.5 cm wide.
- Applicator.
- Scissors.

PROCEDURE
1. Make sure the patient is comfortable, and expose the leg.
2. Cut a length of about 70 cm of elasticated tubular support.
3. Thread the support onto the applicator.
4. Pass the applicator over the foot and position it 3 cm below the knee.
5. Remove the upper end of the elasticated tubular support from the applicator and position it around the leg just below the knee (Figure 15A).
6. Covering the lower leg, ankle, and foot with the elasticated tubular support, slowly remove the applicator towards the foot, leaving the knee and toes exposed (Figure 15B).

Figure 15A

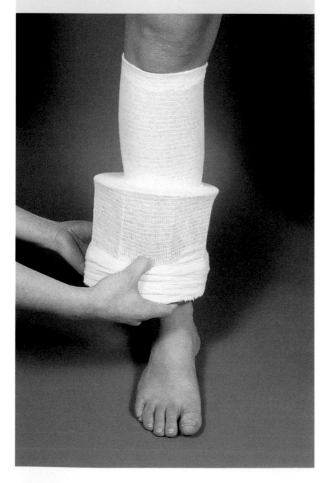

Figure 15B

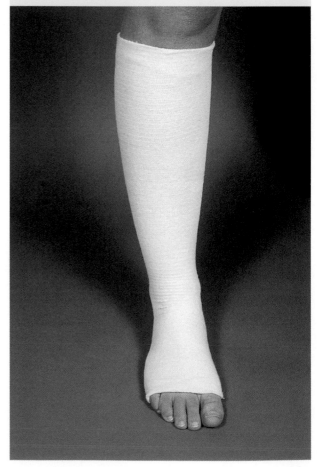

7. If additional support is required, apply a double layer of elasticated tubular support, leaving a 2 cm gap between the two layers to prevent a tourniquet-type effect (Figure 15C).
8. To ensure that the circulation is satisfactory, check the colour and warmth of the foot.

Advice to patients

- Keep the support clean and dry.
- Remove the support for washing the leg and foot, then re-apply; the support can be washed separately.
- Keep the support smooth and remove it at night in order to prevent constriction.
- Follow the **NICER** regimen for acute injuries:
  - **N**: **Non-steroidal anti-inflammatory agents** may be of benefit;
  - **I**: Apply an **Ice** pack to the swollen area for 10 minutes, up to four times daily, and remove the elasticated tubular support before applying the ice pack;
  - **C**: Use the elasticated tubular support for **Compression** and for support for as long as required;
  - **E**: **Elevate** the limb higher than the level of the waist while sitting or lying;
  - **R**: **Rest** or exercise the leg as advised.
- A walking aid may be provided (Procedure 26).

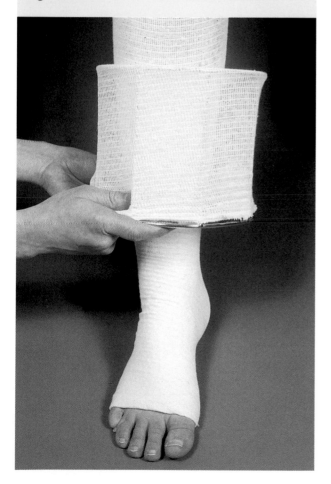

Figure 15C

Crepe bandage to the knee

USES
- Support for sprains or bruises.
- As a pressure dressing, to reduce swelling or prevent bleeding.
- After aspiration of the knee.
- After removal of a plaster of Paris.

EQUIPMENT
- Two crepe bandages, 15 cm wide.
- Elastic adhesive tape, 2.5 cm wide.
- Scissors.

PROCEDURE
1. Make sure the patient is comfortable, and expose the leg.
2. Apply the first crepe bandage in a spiral fashion, from one handspan below the knee to one handspan above the knee.
3. Apply the second crepe bandage in the reverse direction.
4. Secure with elastic adhesive tape (Figures 16A and 16B).

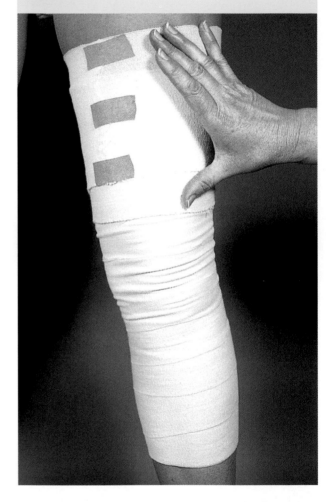

Figure 16A

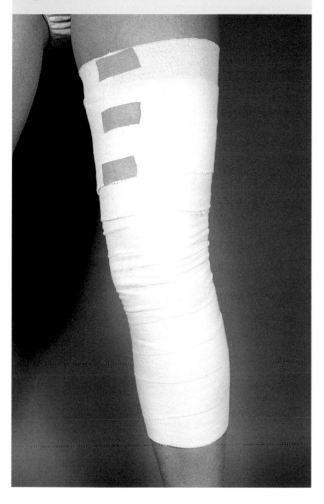

Figure 16B

Advice to patients

- Keep the crepe bandage clean and dry.
- Remove the crepe bandage for washing, then re-apply.
- Follow the **NICER** regimen for acute injuries:

  N: **Non-steroidal anti-inflammatory agents** may be of benefit;

  I: Apply an **Ice** pack to the swollen area for 10 minutes, up to four times daily, and remove the crepe bandage before applying the ice pack;

  C: Use the crepe bandage for **Compression** and for support for as long as required;

  E: **Elevate** the limb higher than the level of the waist while sitting or lying;

  R: **Rest** or exercise the leg as advised. Exercise the quadriceps musculature by holding the foot at a right angle and tightening the muscle at the front of the thigh; raise the straightened leg for five seconds, then lower it slowly; rotate the ankle clockwise and anti-clockwise. Repeat these exercises for five minutes every hour during the day.

- A walking aid may be provided (Procedure 26).

Crepe bandage to the ankle

USES
- Support for sprains or bruises.
- As a pressure dressing, to reduce swelling or prevent bleeding.
- After removal of a plaster of Paris.

EQUIPMENT
- Two crepe bandages, 10 cm wide.
- Elastic adhesive tape, 2.5 cm wide.
- Scissors.

PROCEDURE
1. Make sure the patient is comfortable, and expose the leg.
2. Position the foot at a right angle to the lower leg.
3. Anchor the first crepe bandage around the foot with a fixing turn at the base of the toes.
4. Proceed around the foot in a spiral fashion until the ankle is reached.
5. Use two or three figure-of-eight turns around the ankle.
6. Using the second crepe bandage, continue up the lower leg in a spiral fashion. Cover two-thirds of the width of the bandage with each turn, to about 3 cm below the knee.
7. Ensure that the toes are exposed.
8. Secure with elastic adhesive tape (Figure 17).

Advice to patients

- Keep the crepe bandage clean and dry.
- Remove the crepe bandage for washing, then re-apply.
- Follow the **NICER** regimen for acute injuries:
  N: **Non-steroidal anti-inflammatory agents** may be of benefit;
  I: Apply an **Ice** pack to the swollen area for 10 minutes, up to four times daily, and remove the crepe bandage support before applying the ice pack;
  C: Use the crepe bandage for **Compression** and for support for as long as required;
  E: **Elevate** the limb higher than the level of the waist while sitting or lying;
  R: **Rest** or exercise the leg as advised.
- A walking aid may be provided (Procedure 26).

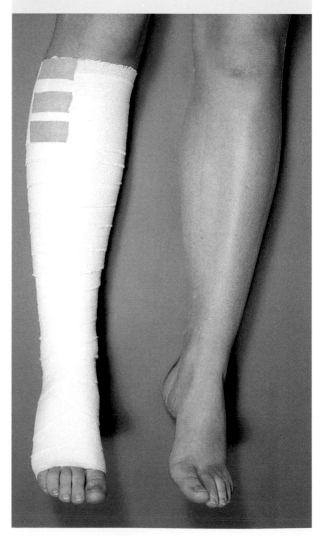

Figure 17

Wool and crepe bandage to the knee

USES
- Injuries of the knee.
- Effusions of the knee.
- After aspiration of the knee.

EQUIPMENT
- Cotton wool roll, 35 cm wide.
- Crepe bandage, 15 cm wide.
- Elastic adhesive tape, 2.5 cm wide.
- Scissors.

PROCEDURE
1. Position the patient on a trolley, ensuring comfort. Expose the knee and place in about 10 degrees of flexion.
2. Apply a layer of cotton wool around the leg from one handspan above the knee to one handspan below the knee (Figure 18A).
3. Cover the cotton wool with the crepe bandage in a spiral fashion up the limb, applying a firm and even pressure.
4. Secure with elastic adhesive tape (Figure 18B).

Advice to patients
- Keep the bandage clean and dry.
- Keeping the bandage on, exercise the ankle and quadriceps musculature by holding the foot at a right angle and tightening the muscle at the front of the thigh; raise the straightened leg for five seconds, then lower it slowly; rotate the ankle clockwise and anti-clockwise. Repeat these exercises for five minutes every hour during the day.
- Use the wool and crepe bandage for as long as advised.
- Elevate the leg when sitting or lying.
- A walking aid may be provided (Procedure 26).

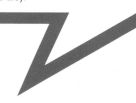

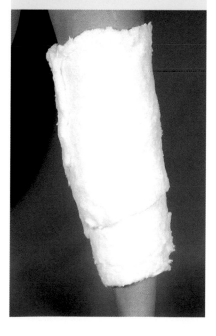

Figure 18A

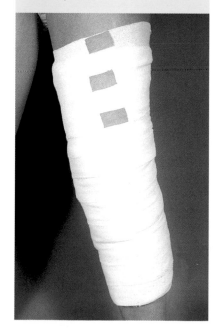

Figure 18B

Wool and crepe bandage to the ankle

USES
- Injuries of the ankle.
- Swelling of the ankle.

EQUIPMENT
- Cotton wool roll, 35 cm wide.
- Two crepe bandages, 10 cm wide.
- Elastic adhesive tape, 2.5 cm wide.
- Scissors.

PROCEDURE
Two people are required for this procedure.
1. Make sure the patient is comfortable, and expose the leg from the knee downwards with the foot supported at a right angle to the lower leg.
2. Apply a layer of cotton wool from the base of the toes to below the knee, overlapping it if necessary (Figure 19A).
3. Starting at the toes and working towards the knee, cover the cotton wool with the crepe bandages in a spiral fashion, applying a firm and even pressure.
4. Secure with elastic adhesive tape (Figure 19B).

Figure 19A

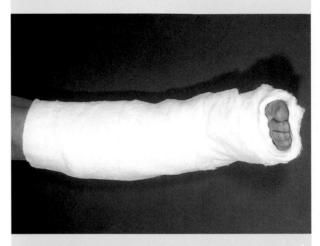

Figure 19B

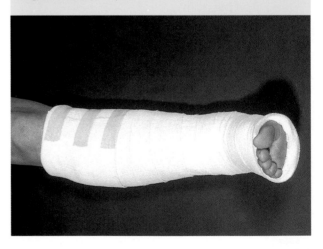

Advice to patients

- Keep the bandage clean and dry.
- Move the knee and toes every hour to reduce stiffness.
- Use the wool and crepe bandage for as long as advised.
- Elevate the leg when sitting or lying.
- A walking aid may be provided (Procedure 26).

Metatarsal brace

USES
- Fractures of the metatarsals or toes.
- Painful conditions of the foot.

EQUIPMENT
- Elasticated metatarsal brace of appropriate size; small, medium, large, or extra large are available.

PROCEDURE
1. Make sure the patient is comfortable, and expose the foot.
2. Place the padded side of the metatarsal brace underneath the foot. The brace may be worn comfortably directly below the fracture or site of pain, or adjacent to it. The patient may adjust the brace to enable comfortable walking on the heel and on the brace.

If additional support is required, the metatarsal brace can be applied over an elasticated tubular support to the ankle (Procedure 15) (Figures 20A and 20B).

Advice to patients

- Keep the brace clean and dry.
- Remove the brace at night, and when resting—it should be worn only for walking.
- Elevate the foot above the level of the waist when sitting or lying, and rest the foot on two pillows at night.
- Exercise the toes by wriggling them.
- Follow advice regarding weightbearing and mobility.
- Use the brace for as long as advised.
- A walking aid may be provided (Procedure 26).

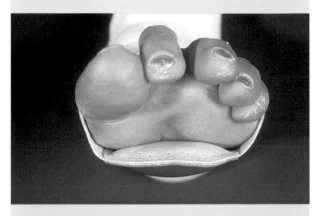

Figure 20A

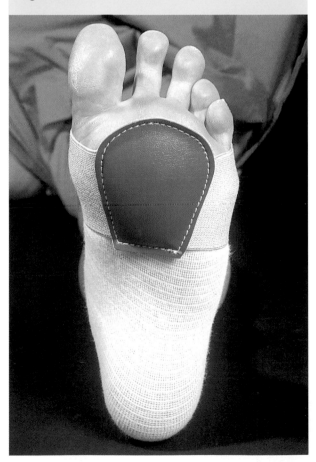

Figure 20B

Toe spica

USES
- Fractures, sprains, or bruises of the great toe.
- After reduction of a dislocated great toe.

EQUIPMENT
- Cotton tubular bandage, 2.5 cm wide.
- Elastic adhesive tape, 2.5 cm wide.
- Scissors.
- Non-allergenic tape (for a patient who is allergic to elastic adhesive tape).

PROCEDURE
1. Ensure that the patient is not allergic to elastic adhesive tape—if the patient is, substitute with a non-allergenic tape.
2. Cut a length of about 8 cm of cotton tubular bandage. Slide it over the great toe and fold back the cut edges, leaving the tip of the toe exposed.
3. Cut about six pieces of elastic adhesive tape of varying lengths from 6 cm to 10 cm.
4. Apply the lengths of elastic adhesive tape from the tip of the toe to the base in a figure-of-eight fashion, forming a 'V' from the nail and over the first metatarsal. Snip the tape as required. Take care not to apply the elastic adhesive tape under tension, as this may restrict the circulation.
5. Complete the spica by applying a length of elastic adhesive tape around the foot to anchor the ends of the tape: leave a 2 cm gap in order to avoid constriction (Figure 21).
6. To ensure that the circulation is satisfactory, check the colour, warmth, and sensation of the great toe, and press its tip to check that the normal colour returns immediately.

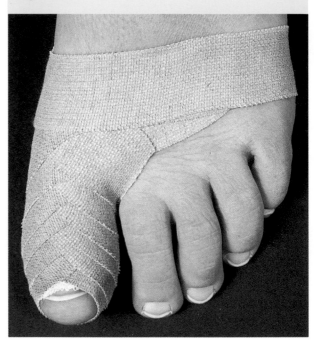

Figure 21

Advice to patients

- Keep the toe spica clean and dry.
- Elevate the foot when sitting or lying.
- If the toe becomes discoloured (other than with delayed bruising) or numb, or severe pain or tingling develop, seek further medical attention.
- Wear the toe spica for as long as advised.

Application of skin extensions

USE
- To provide fixed or balanced traction to the leg, indirectly through the skin, for:
  - Fractured pelvis (particularly central dislocation of the hip).
  - Fractured neck of femur.
  - Fractured shaft of femur (before the application of a Thomas's splint).
  - Fractured tibial plateau.
  - Low back pain.
  - Irritable hip.

EQUIPMENT
- Elastic adhesive tape skin extension (7.5 cm wide) kit, with attached foam padding; various types are available.
- Two cotton conforming bandages, 10 cm wide.
- Elastic adhesive tape, 2.5 cm wide.
- Razor.
- Tincture of benzoin spray.
- Scissors.

PROCEDURE
Two people are required for this procedure. Suitable analgesia is necessary—a femoral nerve block may be useful (Procedure 86).
1. Ensure that the patient is not allergic to elastic adhesive tape—if the patient is, substitute with latex foam rubber skin traction bandage. (This would also be useful for a patient with thin fragile skin.)
2. Reassure the patient and explain the procedure.
3. Make sure the patient is comfortable in a recumbent or semi-recumbent position on a trolley.
4. Expose the leg.
5. Shave the leg from the hip to the ankle on both the inside and the outside of the leg.
6. Spray along both shaved areas with tincture of benzoin; this improves the adhesiveness of the skin extensions.
7. Unroll the elastic adhesive tape skin extensions to the approximate length of the leg.
8. The first person supports the patient's foot and raises the foot about 25 cm from the trolley. A gentle traction on the leg is maintained throughout the procedure to reduce muscular spasm.
9. The second person applies the skin extension on the outside of the leg from above the lateral malleolus up to the greater trochanter. The inside skin extension is then applied from above the medial malleolus up to 5 cm below the groin. Ensure that the foam pieces cover the malleoli on either side of the ankle.
10. Stretch the extensions sideways as they are applied upwards, thus accommodating the contours of the leg and preventing wrinkling. It may be necessary to snip the extensions at the knee in order to accommodate the contours (Figures 22A and 22B).
11. Apply cotton conforming bandages over the extensions, one above and one below the knee, and secure with elastic adhesive tape (Figure 22C).
12. Keep the knee exposed to allow for observation and physiotherapy.
13. Secure the strings to the end of the trolley, maintaining gentle traction—this aids splintage, immobility, and reduction of pain during transportation to the ward.
14. Ensuring maximum comfort, transport the patient to the ward.

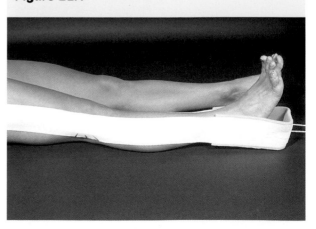

Figure 22A

Figure 22B

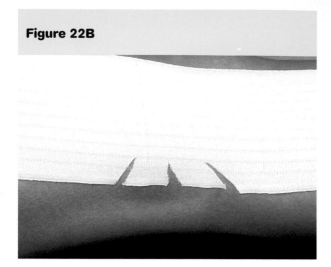

Figure 22C

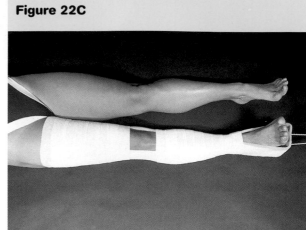

23.

Thomas's splint

USES
- To provide support and/or splintage to a leg after injury.
- To reduce internal blood loss and to relieve pain, particularly after fracture of the shaft of a femur.
- To provide fixed traction, if required.

EQUIPMENT
- Thomas's splint.
- Flannel bandage, 15 cm wide.
- Self-locking safety pins.
- Roll of Gamgee dressing.
- Two calico bandages or two crepe bandages, 15 cm wide.
- Elastic adhesive tape, 2.5 cm wide.
- Tape measure.
- Block.
- Scissors.

PROCEDURE
Four people are required for this procedure. Suitable analgesia is necessary—a femoral nerve block may be useful (Procedure 86).
1. Explain the procedure to the patient. Skin extensions will already have been applied (Procedure 22).
2. Make sure the patient is comfortable in a recumbent or semi-recumbent position, and expose the injured leg.
3. Select the size of the ring of the Thomas's splint by measuring around the thigh of the injured leg at the level of the groin and adding 5 cm in order to allow for swelling. Select the length of the Thomas's splint by measuring the inside of the leg from the groin to the heel and adding 25 cm in order to permit full plantarflexion of the foot.
4. The first person applies gentle traction to the leg by pulling the strings of the skin extensions while simultaneously supporting the heel. Traction is maintained until the procedure is completed.
5. The fracture site is supported by the second person during the application of the splint.
6. The third person carefully passes the splint over the foot and positions it comfortably at the groin.
7. The fourth person cuts the flannel bandage into about six lengths of approximately 60 cm to 90 cm each, according to the size of the splint.

8. Working from the top of the splint down to just above the patient's heel, with a person standing on each side of the trolley, the flannel bandage is threaded around the inner metal bar and both ends are passed under the leg. One person collects the two ends and passes them over the outer bar, under the leg, and back to the other person, who applies cross-traction by ensuring that the flannel slings are taut. Two self-locking safety pins are applied to each sling, underneath the splint, just behind the outer bar (Figure 23A).
9. The whole length of the splint should be lined with a piece of Gamgee dressing. A folded pad of Gamgee dressing is positioned under the knee to ensure that about 10 degrees of flexion is maintained at the joint (Figure 23B).
10. The extension strings are now attached to the end of the Thomas's splint and are tied securely, maintaining gentle traction on the leg.

Figure 23A

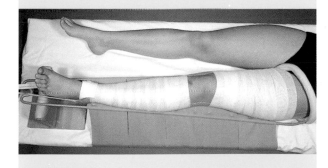

Figure 23B

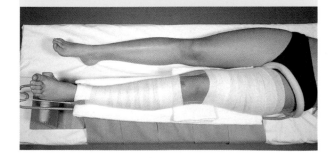

11. The end of the Thomas's splint is supported on a block.
12. Calico bandages or crepe bandages are applied over the splint, incorporating the flannel slings: one is applied from the ankle to below the knee and the other from above the knee to the ring of the splint. These are secured with elastic adhesive tape. The knee should be kept exposed to allow for observation and physiotherapy (Figure 23C).
13. Ensuring maximum comfort, transport the patient to the ward.

Steps 7 to 9 may be performed before the Thomas's splint is applied to the leg.

Figure 23C

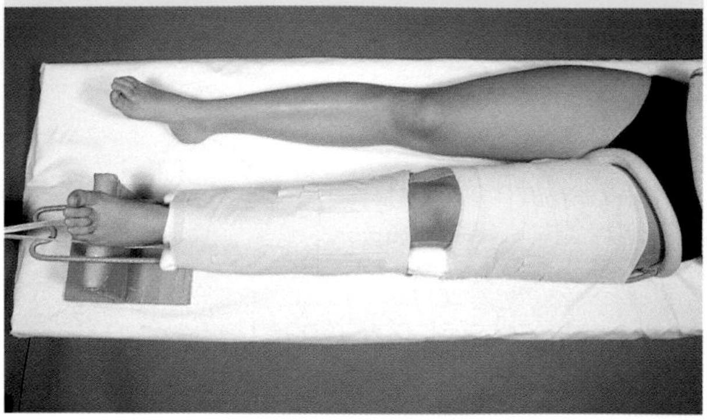

Traction splint

USES
- To provide support and/or splintage to a leg after injury.
- To reduce internal blood loss and to relieve pain, particularly after fracture of the shaft of a femur.
- To aid extrication of a trapped patient following an accident.

EQUIPMENT
- Traction splint: various types are available. Follow the manufacturer's instructions.

PROCEDURE
Two people are required for this procedure. Suitable analgesia is necessary—a femoral nerve block may be useful (Procedure 86).

1. Explain the procedure to the patient. Loosen the locking device and place the splint next to the injured leg, with the ischial pad next to the iliac crest (Figure 24A).
2. Adjust the length of the splint until it extends about 20 cm beyond the patient's heel.
3. Secure the locking device.
4. Open the support straps and locate one at the top of the splint, one above the knee, one below the knee, and one above the ankle.
5. Extend the heel stand.
6. Pull the release ring on the ratchet in order to release the traction strap.
7. Stabilize the limb and check neurovascular function in the leg.
8. An assistant should apply manual traction to the limb and elevate the foot to about 25 cm above the trolley.
9. The assistant maintains traction as the splint is positioned under the limb and aligned with the ischial tuberosity (Figure 24B).
10. Attach the ischial strap across the area of the groin.
11. Attach the ankle hitch (Figure 24C) and insert the 'S' hook into the 'D' ring. Rotate the ratchet in order to apply traction.
12. As the traction is applied, gently lower the limb onto the splint.
13. Apply traction by rotating the ratchet until the patient's pain and muscular spasm are reduced.
14. Secure the remaining straps (Figure 24D) and reassess the neurovascular function in the leg.
15. Ensuring maximum comfort, transport the patient to the ward.

Figure 24A

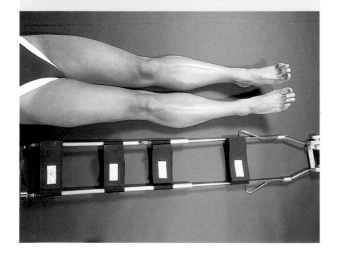

Figure 24B

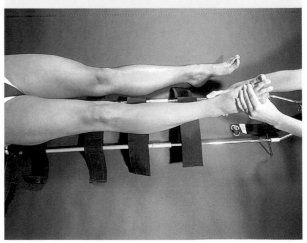

Figure 24C

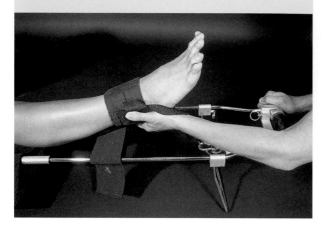

Figure 24D

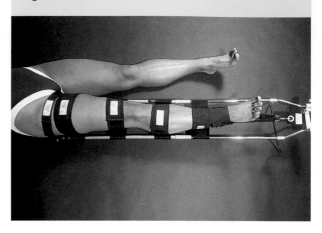

Spinal immobilization using a backboard (including log rolling)

USES
- To immobilize the spine of a patient with suspected spinal injury.
- To aid extrication of a trapped patient following an accident, and transportation.

EQUIPMENT
- Hard cervical collar.
- Long backboard.
- Backboard straps and buckles.
- Two sandbags (or other devices for supporting the head, e.g. foam blocks).
- Elastic adhesive tape, 7.5 cm wide.
- Suction.
- Scissors.

PROCEDURE
Five people are required for this procedure. Suction must be available.

The patient will already have a hard cervical collar in position (Procedure 2). Manual immobilization of the neck must be maintained throughout the procedure.

1. The leader explains the procedure and asks the patient to move the fingers and toes and arms and legs very gently. The leader also tests the patient's sensation to touch.
2. The leader directs the first assistant to place one hand on the patient's shoulder and the other on the patient's elbow, reaching across the patient's chest in doing so.
3. The leader directs the second assistant to place one hand on the patient's forearm and the other under the patient's thigh, reaching over the patient's trunk in doing so.
4. The leader directs the third assistant to place both hands under the patient's far leg, reaching over the patient's near leg in doing so (Figure 25A). In the case of an infant or small child, the second assistant places one hand on either side of the child's pelvis, reaching up from the feet.
5. The leader instructs the team, 'on the count of three', to roll the patient on to his or her side, so that the patient is now facing assistants 1, 2, and 3. The leader ensures continuous alignment of the patient's nose and umbilicus throughout this manoeuvre (Figure 25B).

6. Any loose clothing or debris is removed at this stage and the clinician quickly but carefully examines the patient's back.
7. The fourth assistant is instructed to position the backboard under the patient and to hold it in place.
8. The leader directs the team, 'on the count of three', to roll the patient back on to the backboard.

Figure 25A

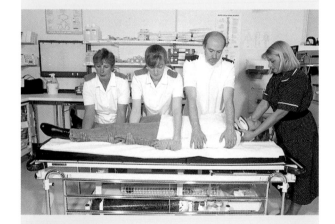

Figure 25B

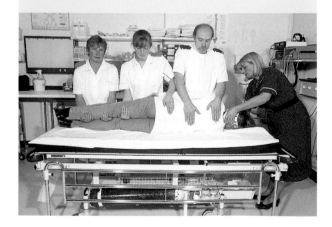

9. Sandbags (or similar devices) are placed on either side of the patient's head. Elastic adhesive tape can be positioned over the forehead and secured to the backboard to prevent movement of the cervical spine.

10. Straps are now placed across the patient's shoulders and hips, and just above the knees (Figure 25C).

11. The leader again asks the patient to move the fingers and toes and arms and legs very gently. The leader again tests the patient's sensation to touch.

12. Manual immobilization of the neck can now be discontinued.

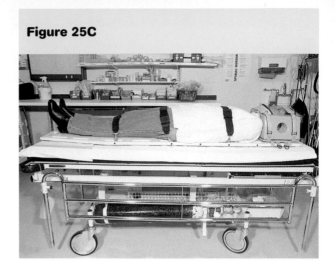

Figure 25C

Walking aids

WALKING STICKS

- With the patient standing upright, and arms by the sides, measure from the wrists to the floor: this is the correct length for the walking stick.
- Ensure that the rubber on the stick has enough tread.
- The stick must always be placed on firm dry ground. Flat shoes should be worn.
- When walking, the stick is held in the hand opposite to the injured leg—it should be held in front of the patient and a little to the side (Figure 26A). The stick is first placed on the ground ahead of the patient, and is followed by the sequence of a small step using the injured leg and a step using the uninjured leg.
- Short steps are used for turning.
- When going upstairs, the stick is held on the side of the injured leg. The first step is taken using the uninjured leg, then the injured leg and the stick are brought up to the same step. The maxim to follow is 'Good leg up first. Bad leg down first'.
- When going downstairs, the stick is held on the side of the injured leg. The first step is taken using the injured leg and the stick together, then the uninjured leg is taken down to the same step. Again, the maxim 'Good leg up first. Bad leg down first' applies.

AXILLARY CRUTCHES

- With the patient standing upright, measure from the axilla to the floor: axillary crutches should be 5 cm shorter than this length.
- Ensure that the rubbers on the axillary crutches have enough tread and that all nuts are tightened.
- The axillary crutches must always be placed on firm dry ground. Flat shoes should be worn.
- The patient's weight is borne by both hands on the handgrips, and not by the axillae.
- The elbows should be slightly flexed (Figure 26B). One axillary crutch should be placed under each axilla and the handgrips should be held firmly. The upper arms are squeezed towards the body in order to hold the crutches firmly. The patient bears weight on one foot,

places the crutches on the floor about 30 cm in front of the feet, and swings the body forwards.

- For partial weightbearing, the majority of the weight is taken by the uninjured leg, and the injured leg is used to maintain balance.
- The patient moves upstairs and downstairs on his or her bottom.
- To sit down, the patient removes the axillary crutches from the axillae and holds them in one hand, using the other hand to steady the seat.

Figure 26A

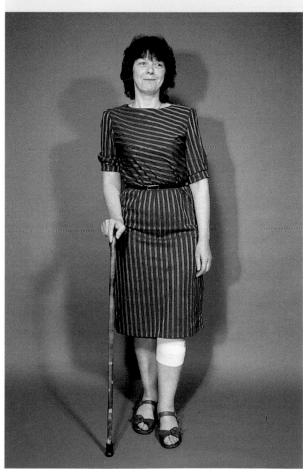

ELBOW CRUTCHES

- With the patient standing upright, and arms by the sides, measure from the wrists to the floor: the handles of elbow crutches should align with the wrists.
- Ensure that the rubbers on the elbow crutches have enough tread.
- The elbow crutches must always be placed on firm dry ground. Flat shoes should be worn.
- Instruct the patient to put both hands through the elbow pieces and take hold of the handles of the crutches. The patient's weight is borne by both hands on the handles and the elbows should be slightly flexed and squeezed into both sides (Figure 26C).
- The injured leg can be held with the knee bent in front or slightly behind the patient's body.
- The patient places the elbow crutches on the floor about 30 cm in front of the feet, and swings the body forwards.

- For partial weightbearing, the majority of the weight is taken by the uninjured leg, and the injured leg is used to maintain balance.
- The patient moves upstairs and downstairs on his or her bottom.
- To sit down or to stand up from sitting, the patient must remove both arms from the elbow crutches and hold the crutches in one hand, using the other hand to steady the seat.

FRAMES

- With the patient standing upright, and arms by the sides, measure from the wrists to the floor: select a frame as near as possible to this height.
- Ensure that the rubbers on the frame have enough tread.
- All four legs of the frame must be placed on firm dry ground. Flat shoes should be worn.

Figure 26B

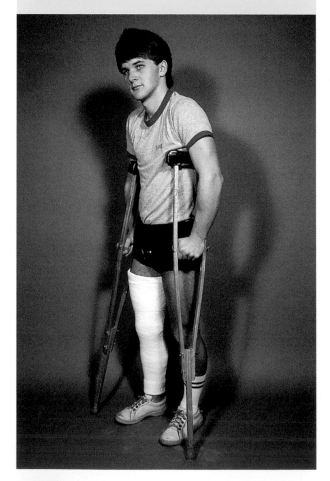

Figure 26C

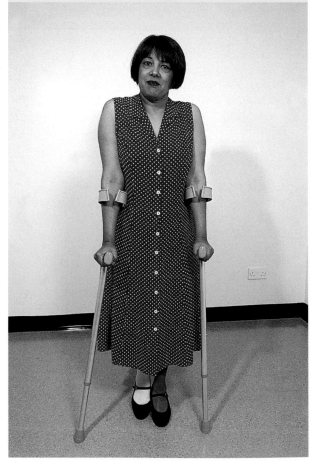

- The patient stands with the frame in front and leans forwards on to the frame, holding the handgrips firmly (Figure 26D).
- For partial weightbearing, the frame is moved slightly forwards, then the injured leg is brought forwards, then the uninjured leg is brought slightly past the injured leg. The arms take the weight of the body.
- The patient must not step too far forwards into the frame because he or she could overbalance.
- For non-weightbearing, the frame is moved slightly forwards and the patient then hops forwards.
- Short steps are used for turning: the frame is moved, then the injured leg, then the uninjured leg.
- The patient moves upstairs and downstairs on his or her bottom.
- To sit down or to stand up from sitting, it is important that the patient does not hold on to the frame but uses the arms of the seat for support. The patient may overbalance if the frame is held on to when sitting down, or if the frame is pulled on when standing up from sitting.

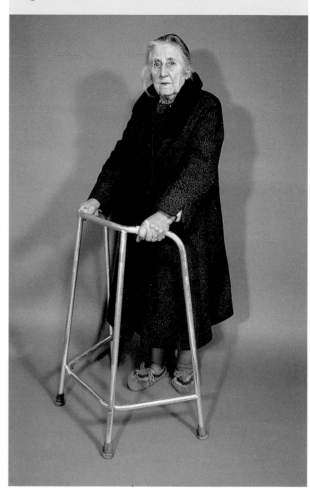

Figure 26D

Plasters

Plaster of Paris is hemihydrated calcium sulphate. When mixed with water, it forms hydrated calcium sulphate and heat is released. Plaster of Paris bandages are available as rolls or slabs. Slabs can be made from rolls by folding the plaster of Paris bandage repeatedly until a slab of suitable thickness is produced. In addition to the traditional plaster of Paris, several types of synthetic casts are available (Figure 27A). Synthetic casts have the advantages of being lighter, stronger, more comfortable, and more radiolucent than traditional plaster of Paris. Synthetic casts also dry more rapidly (usually within about one hour) and do not disintegrate in water. A choice of colours is available for children.

PREPARATION OF THE PATIENT

1. Before applying the plaster, establish how the limb is to be positioned. The patient may be required to sit on a chair or to lie on a trolley or plaster table, depending upon the injured area.
2. Explain the procedure to the patient before applying the plaster.
3. Plasters are often applied while the patient is anaesthetized, after the fracture has been manipulated.
4. For above-elbow or above-knee plasters, or plaster cylinders, expose the entire limb.
5. All jewellery must be removed from the injured limb and must not be replaced while the plaster is in position.
6. When applying the plaster, protect the patient's clothing with a plastic sheet.
7. Any lacerations or abrasions must be cleaned and dressed before cotton tubular bandage or orthopaedic wool is applied; their positions must be noted in case there is leakage from the wound.
8. Particular care must be taken to avoid constriction when a plaster is applied over the elbow or knee.

APPLICATION OF COTTON TUBULAR BANDAGE

Cotton tubular bandage can be pulled onto the limb. This is an optional layer, which often makes the cast tidier and more comfortable.

APPLICATION OF ORTHOPAEDIC WOOL

Orthopaedic wool must be wrapped around the limb smoothly and evenly, avoiding wrinkles. Orthopaedic wool is designed to be eased and stretched around

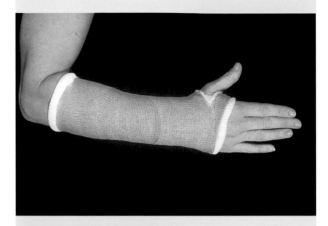

Figure 27A

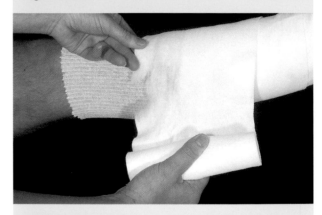

Figure 27B

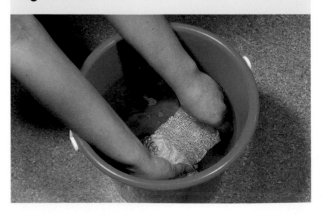

Figure 27C

the body contours and over bony prominences (Figure 27B). Very swollen areas and bony prominences should be protected by a double layer of orthopaedic wool.

APPLICATION OF PLASTER OF PARIS BANDAGES

1. The water to be used should be lukewarm, never hot. The hotter the water, the quicker the plaster sets.
2. Holding the end of the bandage in one hand and the roll of bandage in the other, immerse the bandage in the water until it stops bubbling—usually about five seconds (Figure 27C).
3. Lift out the bandage and squeeze it gently to remove excess water.
4. Apply the bandage around the limb, covering two-thirds of the width of the bandage with each turn (Figure 27D). Smooth it over body contours and bony prominences. It may be necessary to pleat the bandage to do this.
5. The bandages must be applied very carefully and quite quickly, with the position of the limb maintained throughout the procedure. When all the bandages have been applied, the cast can be moulded firmly and smoothly to prevent air from collecting between the layers; trapped air would weaken the plaster.
6. The plaster must be of equal thickness over its entire length; unequal thicknesses would weaken the plaster.
7. A full plaster completely encircles a limb while a plaster slab covers only part of the circumference of a limb; in the former, swelling of the limb is more likely to compromise the circulation. A plaster slab can be removed more rapidly in an emergency.
8. A full plaster may be split (i.e. cut along its full length) immediately after application, using plaster shears. Cut down through the plaster and the orthopaedic wool along the full length of the plaster. Swelling is much less likely to compromise the circulation if the plaster is split; wounds can also be inspected.
9. A full plaster can be bi-valved (i.e. split along both sides). If the top section is removed, a backslab remains and can be secured in position with a crepe bandage. A backslab can also be made directly.

10. Remove any excess plaster from the patient's skin after the procedure.
11. The techniques illustrated may vary in different hospitals, but the practice remains safe as long as the general principles of application are observed.

Figure 27D

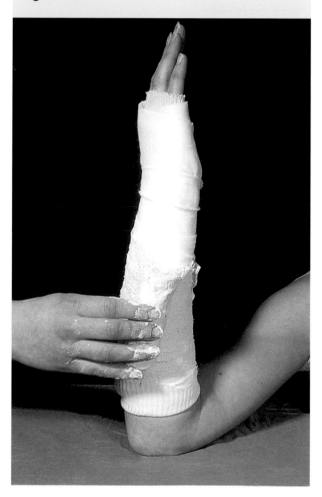

The patient in plaster

EXERCISES
Upper limb

1. Fully straighten out the fingers and thumb (Figure 28A), then make a tight fist and bend the thumb (Figure 28B).
2. Spread the fingers wide apart (Figure 28C), then close them together (Figure 28D).
3. Touch the tip of the thumb to the tip of the little finger (Figure 28E) and slide it down the little finger (Figure 28F).
4. Exercise the shoulder and elbow by removing the arm from the sling, raising both arms above the head (Figure 28G) and circling them to meet behind the back at waist level (Figure 28H).
5. When the plaster is dry, the arm should be used as normally as possible, usually after about 24–48 hours.

Advice to patients

- Return to hospital immediately if the fingers or toes become blue, swollen, very painful, very cold, stiff, red, or begin to tingle.
- Plaster of Paris takes about 48 hours to dry: do not bear weight on the plaster during this time. Modern synthetic casts usually set within about one hour.
- Elevate the arm or leg on a soft surface (e.g. a pillow or a sling) while the plaster is drying.
- If the leg is in plaster, the foot should be higher than the waist when sitting or lying.
- Do not use a hair dryer or direct heat to dry the plaster as this causes crumbling.
- Keep the plaster clean and dry.
- Do not write on a plaster of Paris with a felt-tip pen as it softens the cast.
- Never put anything between the plaster and limb.
- If the plaster cracks or becomes loose, return to hospital.
- Exercise those parts of the limb not included in the plaster. The exercises should be performed for five minutes every hour during the day.

Figure 28A

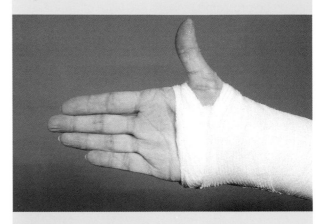

Figure 28B

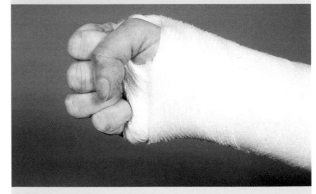

Figure 28C

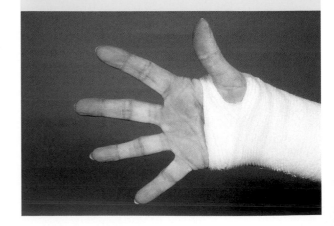

Figure 28D

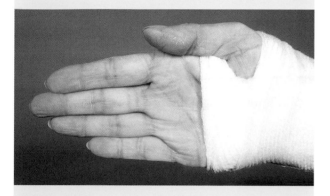

Figure 28E

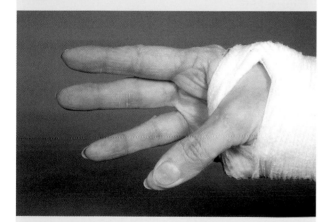

Figure 28F

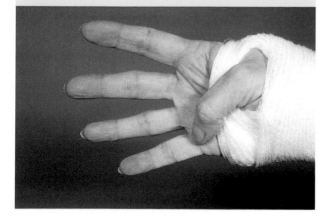

Lower limb

1. Wriggle the toes.
2. Hold the foot at a right angle and tighten the muscle at the front of the thigh.
3. Raise the straightened leg for five seconds, then lower it slowly.
4. Rotate the ankle clockwise and anti-clockwise.

A written information sheet with these instructions and exercises should be given to the patient.

Figure 28G

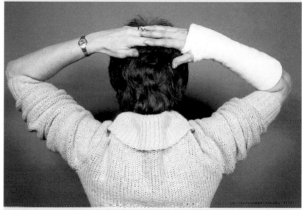

Figure 28H

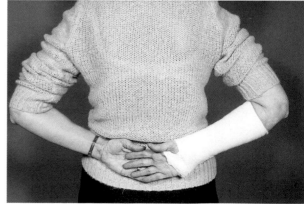

Removal of plasters

PROCEDURE

1. Reassure the patient if using an electric plaster saw as it is noisy and looks dangerous. Ensure that a vacuum device is attached to the electric plaster saw to avoid excessive dust.
2. The blade of an electric plaster saw oscillates forwards and backwards: it does not rotate. It can cut or burn the skin and must be used with care—there should be a layer of orthopaedic wool between the plaster and the skin.
3. Press the blade of the electric plaster saw downwards onto the plaster. When the plaster has been sawn through, a 'give' will be felt. Repeat this action along the entire length of the plaster but avoid the extreme ends, which should be cut with plaster shears. Avoid leaving the electric plaster saw in one place for more than a few seconds as it generates heat. The cutting movement should be up and down and not sideways (Figure 29A).
4. Keep the hands dry when using an electric plaster saw, to avoid an electric shock.
5. Do not use the electric plaster saw near oxygen, as an explosion can occur.
6. When using plaster shears, keep the lower handle parallel to the plaster and move the upper handle up and down (Figure 29B).
7. Push the points of the plaster shears onwards very carefully and, before closing the blades, ensure that they are not going to injure the limb. Particular care is required near joints.
8. If possible, avoid cutting over a bony prominence or a concavity.
9. A plaster on the lower limb can be split along both sides (bi-valved) for easy removal.
10. After being cut along its full length, a plaster of Paris cast on the upper limb can usually be prised open with plaster spreaders. Synthetic casts, however, need to be bi-valved completely before removal.
11. When a plaster has been cut or sawn, the underlying orthopaedic wool and cotton tubular bandage can be cut with blunt-ended bandage scissors ('knobbed scissors') and the plaster removed (Figure 29C).

Modern synthetic casts have to be removed with an electric plaster saw because they are too strong to remove with plaster shears.

Figure 29A

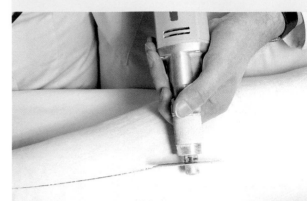

Figure 29B

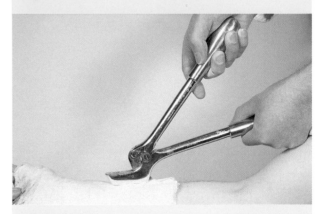

Figure 29C

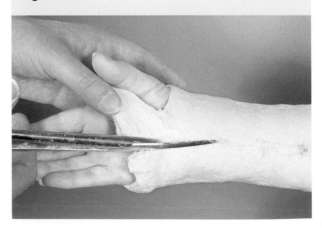

30.

U-slab plaster

USE
- Fracture of the shaft of the humerus.

EQUIPMENT
- Cotton tubular bandage, 10 cm wide.
- Orthopaedic wool, 10 cm wide.
- Plaster of Paris bandage, 15 cm wide.
- Adhesive felt, 5 mm thick.
- Cotton conforming bandage, 15 cm wide.
- Scissors.
- Plastic sheet.
- Bucket of warm water.

PROCEDURE
1. Make sure the patient is comfortable on a chair or trolley, and expose the injured arm fully. The upper arm should hang down in alignment with the body, with the elbow at a right angle and the palm facing the chest. The patient can support the injured arm with the opposite hand.
2. Protect the patient's clothes with the plastic sheet.
3. Apply a length of cotton tubular bandage from below the elbow up to and including the shoulder, snipping the bandage under the axilla for comfort.
4. Make a shoulder pad with the adhesive felt, smoothing this gently from the base of the neck to a little below the tip of the shoulder (Figure 30A).
5. Cover the cotton tubular bandage with orthopaedic wool, extending from 5 cm below the elbow to the tip of the shoulder (Figure 30B).

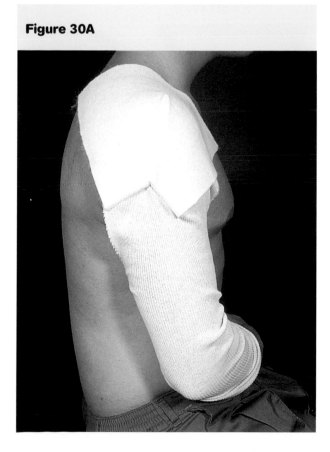

Figure 30A

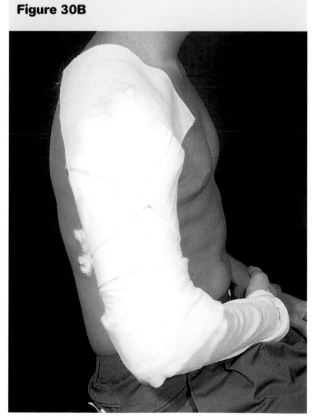

Figure 30B

6. Prepare a plaster of Paris slab of about 10 layers of plaster of Paris bandage. The slab should be long enough to extend from the base of the neck, along the lateral aspect of the upper arm, under the elbow, and up to the axilla. Add 5 cm to allow for shrinkage.

7. Immerse the slab in warm water, holding the ends together to ensure that the layers do not separate.

8. Apply the slab from the axilla down to the elbow, round the elbow, up the lateral aspect of the upper arm, and over the shoulder. Fan the slab over the shoulder padding, moulding it into position to ensure a snug fit (Figure 30C).

9. Smooth out all wrinkles, taking care not to indent the plaster with your fingers.

10. At the shoulder and elbow, turn back the cotton tubular bandage and excess orthopaedic wool over the plaster slab. Ensure that there is no restriction to the circulation at the axilla or elbow.

11. Apply wet cotton conforming bandage in a spiral fashion to anchor the slab in position.

12. Cut a double layer of plaster of Paris bandage, 7.5 cm x 5 cm; immerse it in warm water and use it to anchor the cotton conforming bandage. Apply it over the plaster slab, not over the orthopaedic wool, in order to avoid completing the plaster and thus compromising the circulation.

13. Apply a collar-and-cuff (Procedure 13), allowing the arm to hang and thus bringing the humeral fragments into alignment (Figure 30D).

Figure 30C

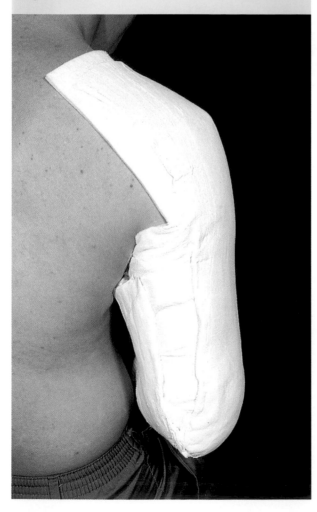

Advice to patients

*   Exercise those parts of the limb not included in the plaster. (Written information and instructions should be provided, as detailed in Procedure 28.)

Figure 30D

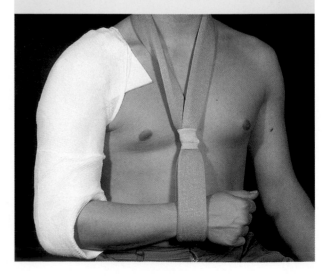

Above-elbow backslab plaster

USES
- Supracondylar fracture of the humerus.
- After reduction of a dislocated elbow.
- Fracture of the head of the radius.
- Fractures of the radius and ulna.

EQUIPMENT
- Cotton tubular bandage, 10 cm wide.
- Orthopaedic wool, 7.5 cm and 10 cm wide.
- Plaster of Paris bandage, 10 cm and 15 cm wide.
- Cotton conforming bandage, 10 cm wide.
- Scissors.
- Plastic sheet.
- Bucket of warm water.

PROCEDURE
1. Make sure the patient is comfortable on a chair or trolley, and expose the injured arm up to the shoulder.
2. Protect the patient's clothes with the plastic sheet.
3. Position the arm with the elbow at a right angle and the hand in a neutral position.
4. Make a plaster of Paris slab by folding the 15 cm wide plaster of Paris bandage five times, so that the final slab extends from the knuckles to the axilla and consists of six layers of plaster of Paris bandage.
5. Cut a semicircle from one corner of the plaster slab to accommodate the thumb.
6. Using the 10 cm wide plaster of Paris bandage, make two slabs about 20 cm in length and five layers thick; these will form the reinforcing supports at the elbow.
7. Snip a 1 cm hole about 5 cm from one end of the cotton tubular bandage. Slide the cotton tubular bandage up the arm to the axilla, putting the patient's thumb through the hole. If the elbow is very swollen or is likely to become increasingly swollen, either omit the cotton tubular bandage or snip a 2 cm piece out of it at the elbow crease.
8. Apply 7.5 cm wide orthopaedic wool from the knuckles to the elbow and 10 cm wide orthopaedic wool from the elbow to the axilla (Figure 31A).
9. Immerse the plaster slab in warm water, holding the ends together to ensure that the layers do not separate.
10. Apply the plaster slab along the posterior surface of the forearm, elbow, and upper arm, from the knuckles to just below the axilla.
11. Immerse the first 20 cm reinforcing slab in warm water and apply it to the medial aspect of the arm, from the proximal forearm to the mid-humerus. Similarly, apply the second 20 cm reinforcing slab to the lateral aspect of the arm in an equivalent position. Take care not to allow the slabs to meet at the elbow crease, as this would complete the plaster and thus compromise the circulation (Figure 31B).

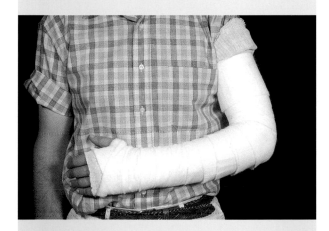

Figure 31A

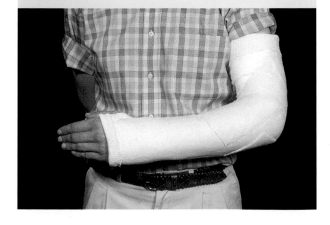

Figure 31B

12. Smooth out all wrinkles, moulding the slab gently to the arm and taking care not to indent the slab with your fingers.

13. Turn back the cotton tubular bandage and excess orthopaedic wool over the plaster slab, ensuring that the knuckles are exposed and that the axilla is free; a couple of small (1 cm) snips in the orthopaedic wool may aid this process.

14. Apply a wet cotton conforming bandage in a spiral fashion to anchor the plaster slab in position, ensuring that the bandage does not constrict the elbow crease.

15. Cut a double layer of plaster of Paris bandage, 7.5 cm x 5 cm; immerse it in warm water and use it to anchor the cotton conforming bandage. Apply it over the plaster slab, not over the orthopaedic wool, in order to avoid completing the plaster and thus compromising the circulation (Figure 31C).

16. Apply a broad arm (triangular) sling (Procedure 11).

The patient may require admission to hospital in order to ensure elevation of the limb, and to observe the peripheral circulation.

Figure 31C

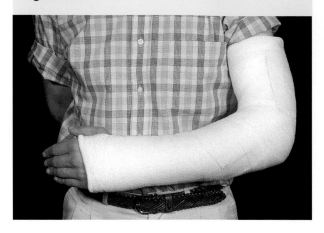

Advice to patients

- Exercise those parts of the limb not included in the plaster. (Written information and instructions should be provided, as detailed in Procedure 28.)

Below-elbow backslab plaster

USES
- Fractures of the distal radius and ulna.
- Certain injuries of the bones or soft tissues of the wrist or hand.
- Inflammation in the area of the wrist or hand (e.g. tenosynovitis).
- After surgery in the area of the wrist or hand (e.g. manipulation of a fracture or repair of a tendon).

EQUIPMENT
- Cotton tubular bandage, 5 cm wide.
- Orthopaedic wool, 7.5 cm wide.
- Plaster of Paris bandage, 15 cm wide.
- Cotton conforming bandage, 10 cm wide.
- Scissors.
- Plastic sheet.
- Bucket of warm water.

PROCEDURE
1. Make sure the patient is comfortable on a chair or trolley, and expose the injured arm to above the elbow.
2. Protect the patient's clothes with the plastic sheet.
3. Position the arm with the wrist and hand in a neutral position, or as indicated according to the specific condition.
4. Make a plaster of Paris slab by folding the plaster of Paris bandage five times so that the final slab extends from the knuckles to 5 cm below the elbow and consists of six layers of plaster of Paris bandage.
5. Round off the corners and cut a semicircle from one corner of the plaster slab to accommodate the thumb (Figure 32A).
6. Snip a small (1 cm) hole about 5 cm from one end of the cotton tubular bandage. Slide the cotton tubular bandage up the arm to the elbow, putting the patient's thumb through the hole.
7. Apply the orthopaedic wool from the knuckles to the elbow, overlapping by half the previous layer and snipping round the thumb to leave it exposed.
8. Make two small (1 cm) snips in the orthopaedic wool at each end, to facilitate the final folding back and edging.
9. Immerse the plaster slab in warm water, holding the ends together to ensure that the layers do not separate.
10. Apply the plaster slab along the posterior surface of the forearm, from the knuckles to just below the elbow.
11. Smooth out all wrinkles, moulding the slab gently to the arm and taking care not to indent the slab with your fingers.
12. Turn back the cotton tubular bandage and excess orthopaedic wool over the plaster slab, ensuring that the knuckles are exposed and that full movement of the elbow is possible (Figures 32B and 32C).

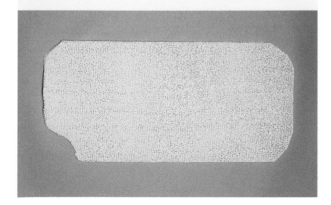

Figure 32A

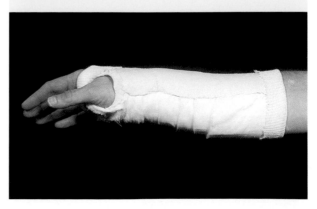

Figure 32B

13. Apply wet cotton conforming bandage in a spiral fashion to anchor the slab in position.
14. Cut a double layer of plaster of Paris bandage, 7.5 cm x 5 cm; immerse it in warm water and use it to anchor the cotton conforming bandage. Apply it over the plaster slab, not over the orthopaedic wool, to avoid completing the plaster and thus compromising the circulation (Figure 32D).
15. Apply a broad arm (triangular) sling (Procedure 11).

Figure 32C

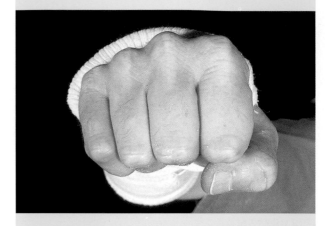

Figure 32D

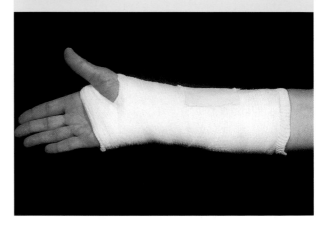

Advice to patients

- Exercise those parts of the limb not included in the plaster. (Written information and instructions should be provided, as detailed in Procedure 28.)

Plaster for Colles' fracture

USE
- Colles' fracture (a fracture of the distal end of the radius in which the distal fragment is angulated posteriorly, displaced posteriorly, and deviated to the radial side, resulting in a 'dinner fork' deformity).

EQUIPMENT
- Cotton tubular bandage, 5 cm wide.
- Orthopaedic wool, 7.5 cm wide.
- Plaster of Paris bandage, 7.5 cm wide.
- Scissors.
- Plastic sheet.
- Bucket of warm water.

PROCEDURE
1. Make sure the patient is comfortable on a chair or trolley, and expose the injured arm to above the elbow.
2. Protect the patient's clothes with the plastic sheet.
3. Position the arm according to the surgeon's instructions; usually the wrist is flexed and in ulnar deviation. The fracture may have been manipulated under Bier's block (intravenous regional anaesthesia) (Procedure 83) or haematoma block (Procedure 84). The surgeon may have to hold the limb in position while the assistant applies the plaster.
4. Snip a small (1 cm) hole about 5 cm from one end of the cotton tubular bandage. Slide the cotton tubular bandage up the arm to the elbow, putting the patient's thumb through the hole.
5. Apply orthopaedic wool from the knuckles to the elbow (Figure 33A).
6. Immerse one roll of plaster of Paris bandage in warm water.
7. Anchor the plaster of Paris bandage around the wrist with two fixing turns. Continue around the hand in a figure-of-eight fashion. Continue up the forearm in a spiral fashion, covering two-thirds of the width of the bandage with each turn, up to the elbow. This usually requires two plaster of Paris bandages.
8. Smooth out all wrinkles and mould the plaster firmly, taking care not to indent the plaster with your fingers.

9. Turn back the cotton tubular bandage and excess orthopaedic wool over the plaster, ensuring that the knuckles and the palmar creases remain exposed and that full movement of the elbow is possible (Figure 33B).
10. Neaten and secure the cotton tubular bandage and excess orthopaedic wool with a strip of plaster of Paris bandage or with a third roll of plaster of Paris bandage (Figures 33C and 33D).
11. Apply a broad arm (triangular) sling (Procedure 11).

Figure 33A

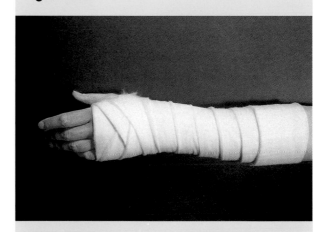

Figure 33B

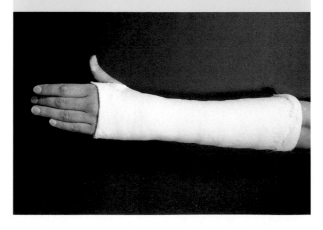

Figure 33C

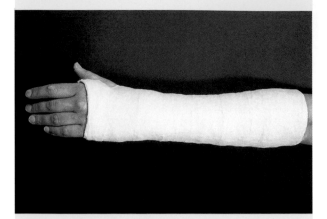

Figure 33D

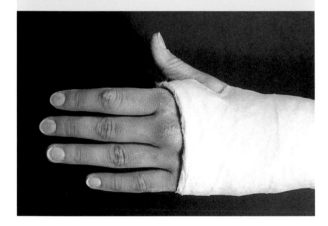

Advice to patients

- Exercise those parts of the limb not included in the plaster. (Written information and instructions should be provided, as detailed in Procedure 28.)

Plaster for Smith's fracture

USE
- Smith's fracture (a fracture of the distal end of the radius in which the distal fragment is angulated anteriorly, displaced anteriorly, and deviated to the radial side).

EQUIPMENT
- Cotton tubular bandage, 5 cm wide.
- Orthopaedic wool, 7.5 cm and 10 cm wide.
- Plaster of Paris bandage, 7.5 cm and 10 cm wide.
- Scissors.
- Plastic sheet.
- Bucket of warm water.

PROCEDURE
1. Make sure the patient is comfortable on a chair or trolley, and expose the injured arm to the shoulder.
2. Protect the patient's clothes with the plastic sheet.
3. Snip a small (1 cm) hole about 5 cm from one end of the cotton tubular bandage. Slide the cotton tubular bandage up the arm to the axilla, putting the patient's thumb through the hole.
4. The arm is positioned according to the surgeon's instructions; usually the forearm is fully supinated, the wrist extended, and the elbow at a right angle.
5. Apply 7.5 cm wide orthopaedic wool from the knuckles to the elbow and 10 cm wide orthopaedic wool from the elbow to the axilla (Figure 34A).
6. Immerse one roll of 7.5 cm wide plaster of Paris bandage in warm water.
7. Anchor the plaster of Paris bandage around the wrist with two fixing turns. Continue around the hand in a figure-of-eight fashion. Continue up the forearm in a spiral fashion, covering two-thirds of the width of the bandage with each turn, up to the elbow. Ensure that the thumb is exposed.
8. Repeat steps 6 and 7 with a second roll of 7.5 cm wide plaster of Paris bandage (Figure 34B).
9. Immerse one roll of 10 cm wide plaster of Paris bandage in warm water.
10. Apply the plaster of Paris bandage from below the elbow to the axilla, covering two-thirds of the width of the bandage with each turn.
11. Repeat steps 9 and 10 with a second roll of 10 cm wide plaster of Paris bandage.
12. Smooth out all wrinkles and mould the plaster firmly, taking care not to indent the plaster with your fingers.
13. Turn back the cotton tubular bandage and excess orthopaedic wool over the plaster, ensuring that the knuckles, thumb, and axilla remain exposed (Figures 34C and 34D).
14. Neaten and secure the edges with a strip of plaster of Paris bandage (Figure 34E).
15. Apply a broad arm (triangular) sling (Procedure 11).

Figure 34A

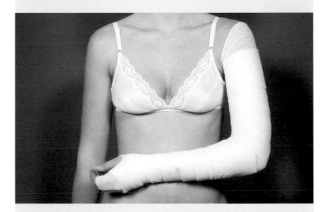

Figure 34B

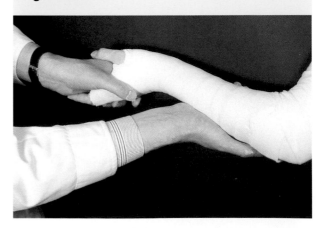

Figure 34C

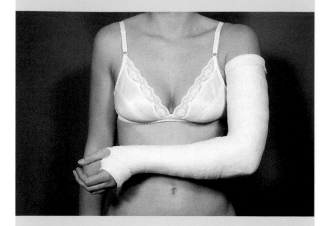

Figure 34D

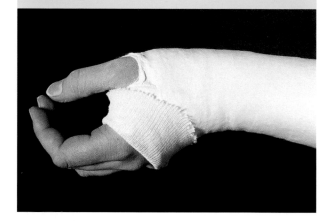

Figure 34E

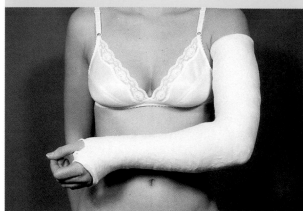

Advice to patients

- Exercise those parts of the limb not included in the plaster. (Written information and instructions should be provided, as detailed in Procedure 28.)

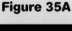

Plaster for a fracture of the scaphoid bone

USES
- Fracture of the scaphoid bone.
- Suspected fracture of the scaphoid bone.

EQUIPMENT
- Cotton tubular bandage, 1.5 cm and 5 cm wide.
- Orthopaedic wool, 7.5 cm wide.
- Plaster of Paris bandage, 7.5 cm wide.
- Scissors.
- Plastic sheet.
- Bucket of warm water.

PROCEDURE
1. Make sure the patient is comfortable, and expose the injured arm to above the elbow with the elbow resting on a table.
2. Protect the patient's clothes with the plastic sheet.
3. Snip a small (1 cm) hole about 5 cm from one end of the 5 cm wide cotton tubular bandage. Slide the 5 cm wide cotton tubular bandage up the arm to the elbow, putting the patient's thumb through the hole.
4. Apply a length of 1.5 cm wide cotton tubular bandage to the thumb.
5. The arm is positioned according to local policy, as surgeons have different opinions. The position described and illustrated here is the most common position selected. Ask the patient to cock back the wrist and to hold an imaginary roll of bandage in the palm of the hand, with the tip of the index finger touching the tip of the thumb. This position must be maintained until the plaster is completed (Figures 35A and 35B).

Figure 35A

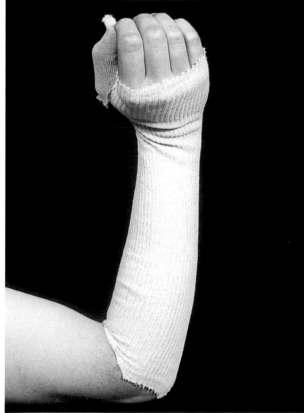

Figure 35B

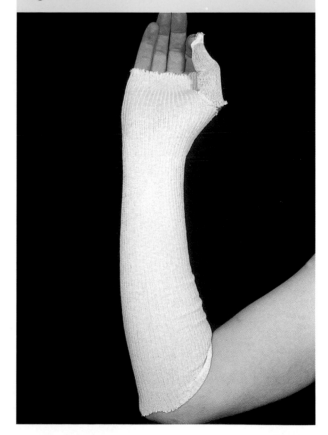

6. Apply orthopaedic wool from the knuckles to the elbow and around the thumb, snipping the orthopaedic wool in order to ease the fit (Figure 35C).
7. Immerse one roll of plaster of Paris bandage in warm water and apply this from just below the elbow, working in a spiral fashion towards the wrist. Two-thirds of the width of the bandage should be covered with each turn. Aim to include the wrist and the thumb with this first roll, so that the plaster of Paris bandage is applied around the thumb to the interphalangeal joint, and around the hand to the knuckles and the palmar crease. The bandage may be snipped around the web space of the thumb in order to minimize the thickness around this area.
8. Immerse another roll of plaster of Paris bandage in warm water and apply this on top of the first application. Do not attempt to smooth the bandage between the layers as this will weaken the final cast.
9. Smooth out all wrinkles and mould the plaster firmly, taking care not to indent the plaster with your fingers.
10. Turn back the cotton tubular bandage and excess orthopaedic wool over the plaster, ensuring that the knuckles, palmar crease, distal half of the thumb, and elbow remain exposed.
11. Neaten and secure the edges with a strip of plaster of Paris bandage (Figures 35D and 35E).
12. Apply a broad arm (triangular) sling (Procedure 11).

Figure 35C

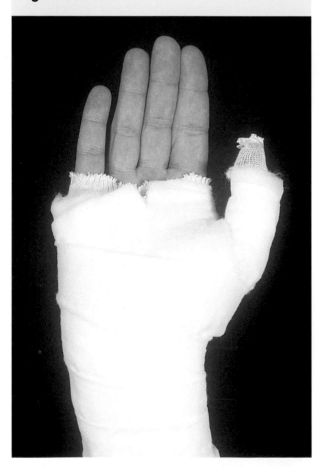

Figure 35D

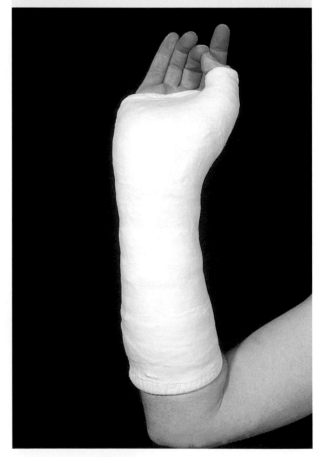

Figure 35E

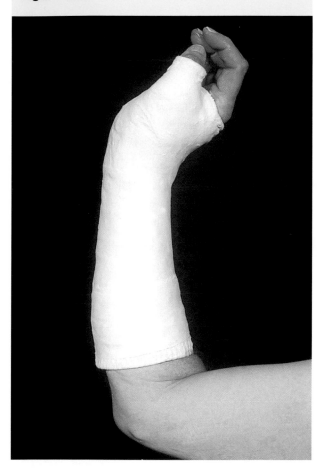

Advice to patients

- Exercise those parts of the limb not included in the plaster. (Written information and instructions should be provided, as detailed in Procedure 28.)

Plaster for Bennett's fracture

USE
- Bennett's fracture (a fracture–dislocation of the first carpometacarpal joint at the base of the thumb).

EQUIPMENT
- Cotton tubular bandage, 1.5 cm and 5 cm wide.
- Orthopaedic wool, 7.5 cm wide.
- Plaster of Paris bandage, 10 cm wide.
- Adhesive felt, 1 cm thick.
- Scissors.
- Plastic sheet.
- Bucket of warm water.

PROCEDURE
1. Make sure that the patient is comfortable on a chair, and expose the injured arm to above the elbow with the elbow resting on a table.
2. Protect the patient's clothes with the plastic sheet.
3. Position the arm with the wrist in slight dorsiflexion. Traction should be applied to the thumb, and the thumb should be in abduction with pressure applied to the lateral aspect of the base of the first metacarpal. Local policy may necessitate a variation of this position.
4. Apply 5 cm wide cotton tubular bandage to the forearm and 1.5 cm wide cotton tubular bandage to the thumb.
5. Place the adhesive felt (cut to about 3 cm square) over the cotton tubular bandage over the base of the first metacarpal (Figures 36A and 36B).
6. Apply orthopaedic wool from the elbow to the knuckles and around the thumb, snipping the orthopaedic wool as necessary.
7. Immerse one roll of plaster of Paris bandage in warm water and apply this from just below the elbow to the hand, working in a spiral fashion.

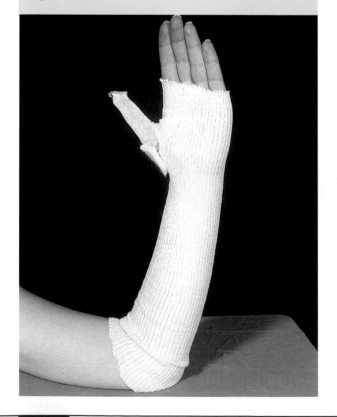

Figure 36A

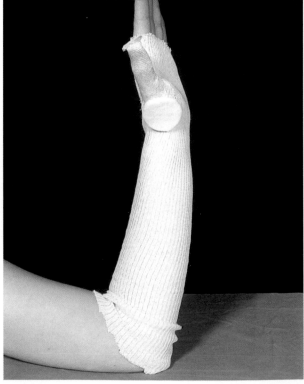

Figure 36B

Two-thirds of the width of the bandage should be covered with each turn. The plaster should finish just below the knuckles, and the palmar crease should be exposed. The plaster should include the thumb, leaving the tip of the thumb exposed.

8. Immerse a second roll of plaster of Paris bandage in warm water and apply this on top of the first application.
9. Smooth out all wrinkles and mould the plaster firmly, taking care not to indent the plaster with your fingers. Light traction should be applied to the thumb while the plaster sets (Figure 36C).
10. Turn back the cotton tubular bandage and excess orthopaedic wool over the plaster.
11. Neaten and secure the edges with a strip of plaster of Paris bandage (Figure 36D).

12. Apply a broad arm (triangular) sling (Procedure 11).
13. X-rays will be required to ensure that a satisfactory reduction has been achieved and maintained.

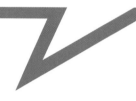

Advice to patients

- Exercise those parts of the limb not included in the plaster. (Written information and instructions should be provided, as detailed in Procedure 28.)

Figure 36C

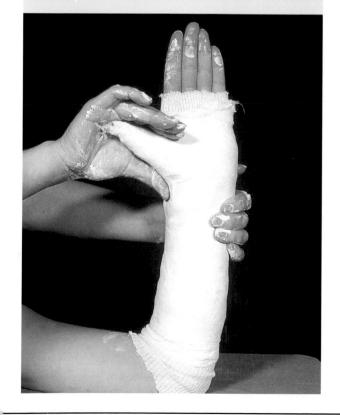

Figure 36D

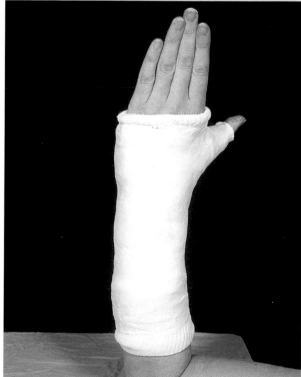

Plaster cylinder

USES
- Fracture of the patella.
- After reduction of a dislocated patella.
- Certain soft tissue injuries of the knee.
- Fracture of the tibial plateau.

EQUIPMENT
- Cotton tubular bandage, 10 cm wide.
- Orthopaedic wool, 10 cm and 15 cm wide.
- Plaster of Paris bandage, 15 cm and 20 cm wide.
- Adhesive felt, 1 cm thick.
- Scissors.
- Plastic sheet.
- Bucket of warm water.
- Plaster bridge.

PROCEDURE
Two people are required for this procedure.
1. Make sure the patient is comfortable on a plaster table, and expose the injured leg to the groin with the knee supported by the plaster bridge when necessary, at an angle of about 10 degrees of flexion.
2. Protect the patient's clothes with the plastic sheet.
3. One person keeps the leg raised by holding the foot.
4. Apply the cotton tubular bandage from the ankle to the groin.
5. Cut a piece of adhesive felt about 7.5 cm wide and long enough to encircle the ankle. Apply this just above the malleoli, encircling the ankle in order to help to prevent the plaster cylinder from slipping down the leg (Figure 37A).
6. Apply 10 cm wide orthopaedic wool from above the malleoli to the knee, and 15 cm wide orthopaedic wool from the knee to the groin, snipping it as necessary in order to allow it to conform to the shape of the limb.
7. Immerse one roll of 15 cm wide plaster of Paris bandage in warm water and apply this in a spiral fashion from above the malleoli to the knee. Two-thirds of the width of the bandage should be covered with each turn. Repeat this procedure with a second roll of 15 cm wide plaster of Paris bandage.
8. The plaster bridge is now removed and one person maintains the knee in the required position throughout the remainder of

Figure 37A

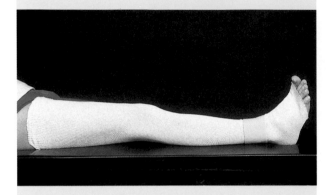

Figure 37B

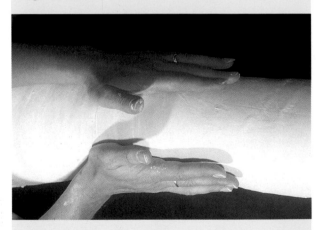

Figure 37C

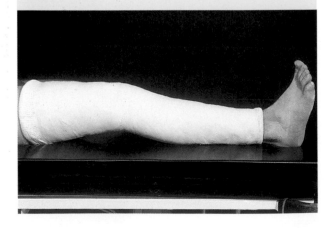

the procedure, usually at an angle of about 10 degrees of flexion.

9. Immerse a third roll of 15 cm wide plaster of Paris bandage in warm water and apply this in a spiral fashion from below the knee to the mid-thigh. Repeat this procedure with a fourth roll of 15 cm wide plaster of Paris bandage.

10. Immerse a fifth roll of 15 cm wide plaster of Paris bandage in warm water and apply this in a spiral fashion from the mid-thigh to the groin. Repeat this procedure with a sixth roll of 15 cm wide plaster of Paris bandage.

11. Mould the plaster cylinder with the palms of your hands on the medial and lateral aspects of the thigh, just above and around the knee, in order to help to prevent the plaster cylinder from slipping down the leg (Figure 37B).

12. Smooth out all wrinkles and mould the plaster firmly, taking care not to indent the plaster with your fingers.

13. Turn back the cotton tubular bandage and excess orthopaedic wool over the plaster cylinder, ensuring that full movements of the hip and ankle are possible.

14. Neaten the plaster cylinder with a roll of 20 cm wide plaster of Paris bandage, applied over the full length of the cylinder in a spiral fashion, securing the cotton tubular bandage and excess orthopaedic wool at the edges (Figure 37C). Alternatively, the cotton tubular bandage and excess orthopaedic wool can be turned back and anchored with two plaster of Paris strips at the upper and lower edges of the plaster cylinder, thus reducing the weight of the plaster cylinder and helping to prevent it from slipping down the leg.

Advice to patients

- Exercise those parts of the limb not included in the plaster. (Written information and instructions should be provided, as detailed in Procedure 28.)
- Use the walking aid provided (Procedure 26).

Above-knee backslab plaster

USE
- Fractures of the tibia and fibula, above the lower quarter. A plaster of Paris backslab is applied in order to provide temporary splintage in the presence of swelling or before or after manipulation of a fracture.

EQUIPMENT
- Cotton tubular bandage, 10 cm wide.
- Orthopaedic wool, 15 cm wide.
- Plaster of Paris bandage slab, 20 cm wide.
- Cotton conforming bandage, 10 cm wide.
- Scissors.
- Plastic sheet.
- Bucket of warm water.
- Plaster bridge.

PROCEDURE
Two or three people are required for this procedure.
1. Make sure the patient is comfortable on a plaster table, and expose the injured leg to the groin with the knee supported by the plaster bridge when necessary, at an angle of about 10 degrees of flexion.
2. Protect the patient's clothes with the plastic sheet.
3. One person holds the foot at a right angle throughout the procedure.
4. Apply the cotton tubular bandage from the toes to the groin.
5. Apply orthopaedic wool from the toes to the groin (Figure 38A).
6. Cut a plaster of Paris bandage slab to extend from the base of the toes, along the back of the lower leg and knee, and along the back of the thigh almost to the buttock.
7. Immerse the plaster of Paris bandage slab in warm water, holding the ends together to ensure that the layers do not separate.
8. With the knee at an angle of about 10 degrees of flexion, apply the plaster of Paris bandage slab from the base of the toes, underneath the heel, along the posterior surface of the lower leg and the knee, and as high up the posterior surface of the thigh as is comfortable for the patient (Figure 38B).
9. If the patient has a large leg, it may be necessary to strengthen the backslab by using additional layers of plaster of Paris

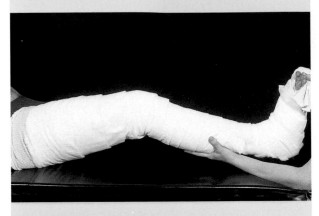

Figure 38A

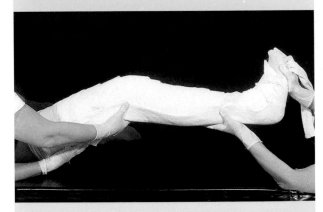

Figure 38B

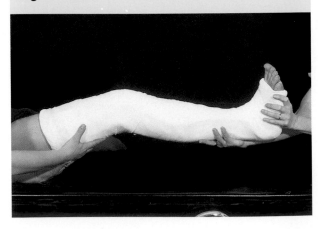

Figure 38C

bandage slab along the inner and outer aspects of the leg.

10. Smooth out all wrinkles, taking care not to indent the plaster with your fingers.

11. Turn back the cotton tubular bandage and excess orthopaedic wool over the plaster slab, ensuring that the groin and toes are exposed.

12. Apply wet cotton conforming bandage in a spiral fashion to anchor the plaster of Paris bandage slab in position.

13. Cut a double layer of plaster of Paris bandage, 7.5 cm x 5 cm; immerse it in warm water and use it to anchor the cotton conforming bandage. Apply it over the plaster of Paris slab, not over the orthopaedic wool, in order to avoid completing the plaster and thus compromising the circulation (Figure 38C).

Advice to patients

- Exercise those parts of the limb not included in the plaster. (Written information and instructions should be provided, as detailed in Procedure 28.)
- Use the walking aid provided (Procedure 26).

Above-knee plaster

USE
- Fractures of the tibia and fibula, above the lower quarter.

EQUIPMENT
- Cotton tubular bandage, 10 cm wide.
- Orthopaedic wool, 10 cm and 15 cm wide.
- Plaster of Paris bandage, 15 cm and 20 cm wide.
- Scissors.
- Plastic sheet.
- Bucket of warm water.
- Plaster bridge.

PROCEDURE
Three people are required for this procedure.

1. Make sure the patient is comfortable on a plaster table, and expose the injured leg to the groin with the knee supported by the plaster bridge when necessary, at an angle of about 10 degrees of flexion.
2. Protect the patient's clothes with the plastic sheet.
3. One person holds the foot at a right angle throughout the procedure.
4. Apply the cotton tubular bandage from the toes to the groin (Figure 39A).
5. Apply 10 cm wide orthopaedic wool from the toes to the knee and 15 cm wide orthopaedic wool from the knee to the groin.
6. Immerse one roll of 15 cm wide plaster of Paris bandage in warm water and apply this from the base of the toes to the ankle. Repeat this procedure with a second roll of 15 cm wide plaster of Paris bandage.
7. Immerse a third roll of 15 cm wide plaster of Paris bandage in warm water and apply this in a spiral fashion from the ankle to the knee, pleating it where necessary to accommodate the contours of the limb. Two-thirds of the width of the bandage should be covered with each turn. Repeat this procedure with a fourth roll of 15 cm wide plaster of Paris bandage (Figure 39B). Never attempt to plaster both the ankle and the knee in one application. Always stabilize the fracture first with the below-knee section of the plaster and then proceed as follows.
8. The plaster bridge is now removed and one person maintains the knee at an angle of about

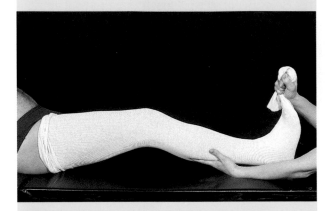

Figure 39A

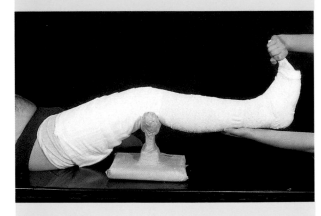

Figure 39B

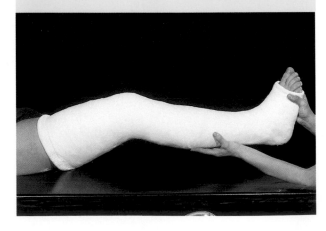

Figure 39C

10 degrees of flexion throughout the remainder of the procedure.

9. Immerse a fifth roll of 15 cm wide plaster of Paris bandage in warm water and apply this in a spiral fashion from below the knee to the mid-thigh. Repeat this procedure with a sixth roll of 15 cm wide plaster of Paris bandage.

10. Immerse one roll of 20 cm wide plaster of Paris bandage in warm water and apply this in a spiral fashion from above the knee to the groin. Repeat this procedure with a second roll of 20 cm wide plaster of Paris bandage.

11. Smooth out all wrinkles and mould the plaster firmly, taking care not to indent the plaster with your fingers.

12. Turn back the cotton tubular bandage and excess orthopaedic wool over the plaster, ensuring that the groin and toes remain exposed.

13. Neaten and bond the two sections of plaster with one or two more plaster of Paris bandages, applied along the full length of the leg from the toes to the groin in a spiral fashion, securing the cotton tubular bandage and excess orthopaedic wool at the edges (Figure 39C).

Advice to patients

- Exercise those parts of the limb not included in the plaster. (Written information and instructions should be provided, as detailed in Procedure 28.)
- Use the walking aid provided (Procedure 26).

Below-knee backslab plaster

USES
- Fractures of the fibula.
- Certain fractures around the ankle.
- Certain sprains of the ankle.
- Certain fractures of the bones of the foot.

A plaster of Paris backslab is applied in order to provide temporary splintage in the presence of swelling or before or after manipulation of a fracture.

EQUIPMENT
- Cotton tubular bandage, 7.5 cm wide.
- Orthopaedic wool, 10 cm wide.
- Plaster of Paris bandage slab, 15 cm wide.
- Cotton conforming bandage, 10 cm wide.
- Scissors.
- Plastic sheet.
- Bucket of warm water.
- Plaster bridge.

PROCEDURE
Two people are required for this procedure.
1. Make sure the patient is comfortable on a plaster table, and expose the injured leg to the thigh with the knee supported by the plaster bridge when necessary.
2. Protect the patient's clothes with the plastic sheet.
3. One person holds the foot at a right angle throughout the procedure.
4. Apply the cotton tubular bandage from the toes to the knee (Figure 40A).
5. Apply orthopaedic wool from the toes to the knee.
6. Cut a plaster of Paris bandage slab to extend from the base of the toes, along the back of the lower leg, to just below the knee.
7. Immerse the plaster of Paris bandage slab in warm water, holding the ends together to ensure that the layers do not separate.
8. Apply the plaster of Paris bandage slab from the base of the toes, underneath the heel, and along the posterior surface of the lower leg to about 5 cm below the knee (Figure 40B).
9. Smooth out all wrinkles, taking care not to indent the plaster with your fingers.
10. Turn back the cotton tubular bandage and excess orthopaedic wool over the plaster slab, ensuring that the toes are exposed and that the patient can flex the knee.

Figure 40A

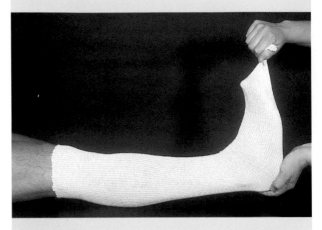

Figure 40B

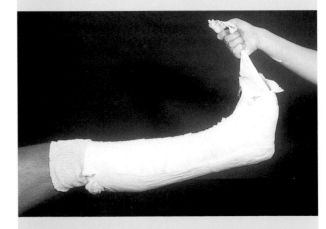

Figure 40C

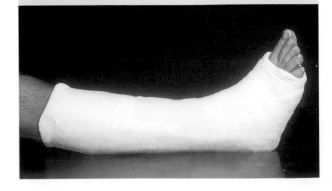

11. Apply wet cotton conforming bandage in a spiral fashion to anchor the plaster of Paris bandage slab in position.
12. Cut a double layer of plaster of Paris bandage, 7.5 cm x 5 cm; immerse it in warm water and use it to anchor the cotton conforming bandage. Apply it over the plaster of Paris bandage slab, not over the orthopaedic wool, in order to avoid completing the plaster and thus compromising the circulation (Figure 40C).

Advice to patients

- Exercise those parts of the limb not included in the plaster. (Written information and instructions should be provided, as detailed in Procedure 28.)
- Use the walking aid provided (Procedure 26).

Below-knee plaster

USES
- Fractures of the fibula.
- Certain fractures around the ankle.
- Certain sprains of the ankle.
- Certain fractures of the bones of the foot.

EQUIPMENT
- Cotton tubular bandage, 7.5 cm wide.
- Orthopaedic wool, 10 cm wide.
- Plaster of Paris bandage, 15 cm wide.
- Scissors.
- Plastic sheet.
- Bucket of warm water.
- Plaster bridge.

PROCEDURE
Two people are required for this procedure.
1. Make sure the patient is comfortable on a plaster table, and expose the injured leg to the thigh with the knee supported by the plaster bridge when necessary.
2. Protect the patient's clothes with the plastic sheet.
3. One person holds the foot at a right angle throughout the procedure.
4. Apply the cotton tubular bandage from the toes to the knee.
5. Apply orthopaedic wool from the toes to the knee, snipping the orthopaedic wool as necessary in order to allow it to conform to the contours of the leg.
6. Immerse one roll of plaster of Paris bandage in warm water and apply this from the base of the toes to the ankle. Repeat this procedure with a second roll of plaster of Paris bandage.
7. Immerse a third roll of plaster of Paris bandage in warm water and apply this in a spiral fashion from the ankle to the knee. Two-thirds of the width of the bandage should be covered with each turn. Repeat this procedure with a fourth roll of plaster of Paris bandage (Figure 41A).

Steps 8, 9 and 10 are omitted if a non-weightbearing plaster is required.
8. Make a plaster of Paris foot-piece slab by folding the plaster of Paris bandage seven times, so that the final slab is the length of the foot and consists of eight layers of plaster of Paris bandage.
9. Immerse the plaster foot-piece slab in warm water, holding the ends together to ensure that the layers do not separate.
10. Apply the plaster foot-piece slab from the base of the toes to the heel and smooth it into position.
11. Smooth out all wrinkles and mould the plaster firmly, taking care not to indent the plaster with your fingers.

Figure 41A

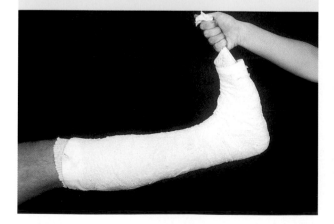

Figure 41B

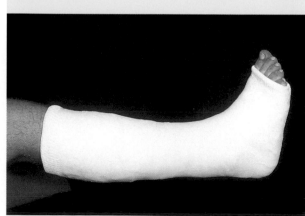

12. Turn back the cotton tubular bandage and excess orthopaedic wool over the plaster, ensuring that the toes remain exposed and that full movement of the knee is possible.
13. Neaten the plaster with a final roll of plaster of Paris bandage, applied in a spiral fashion from the toes to about 5 cm below the knee, securing the foot-piece slab and the cotton tubular bandage and excess orthopaedic wool at the edges (Figure 41B). Alternatively, if the foot-piece slab is not required (because the plaster is a non-weightbearing one), the cotton tubular bandage and excess orthopaedic wool can be turned back and anchored with plaster of Paris strips at the toes and knee.

If a synthetic cast (other than plaster of Paris) is used, the supporting foot-piece slab is not necessary because the cast is of sufficient strength to allow weightbearing.

Advice to patients

- Exercise those parts of the limb not included in the plaster. (Written information and instructions should be provided, as detailed in Procedure 28.)
- Use the walking aid provided (Procedure 26).

Wound irrigation and cleansing (wound toilet)

USE
• To clean a wound.

In an emergency department, the nature of an injury may prevent the use of a strict aseptic technique. However, all wounds must be cleansed and debrided as thoroughly as possible. Local anaesthesia is sometimes required to allow adequate wound toilet.

EQUIPMENT
• Sterile dressing pack, including:
  Tray or receiver.
  Gauze.
  Gloves.
  Towels.
  Gallipot.
• Cleansing solution (e.g. sterile normal saline).
• Sterile 10 ml syringe.
• Sterile forceps.
• Sterile scissors.

PROCEDURE
Sterile gloves are worn throughout the procedure.
1. Explain the procedure to the patient.
2. Make sure the patient is comfortable, and expose the injured area.
3. Local anaesthesia may be required.
4. Fill the syringe with cleansing solution and gently squirt the solution into the wound (Figure 42).

Work away from clean areas and towards dirty areas, to avoid contaminating the clean areas.
5. It may be necessary to remove debris (e.g. grit) from the wound by picking it out with sterile forceps. Any necrotic tissue must be removed with sterile scissors.
6. According to the nature of the wound, it may now be dressed or sutured, or skin-closure strips applied.

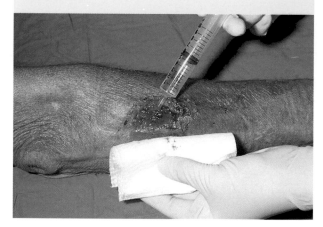

Figure 42

43.

Dry dressing

USE
- To protect a broken skin surface.

EQUIPMENT
- Non-adherent absorbent dressing (or an alternative adhesive dressing).
- Permeable adhesive tape, 1.25 cm wide.
- Gauze.
- Cotton conforming bandage.
- Elastic adhesive tape, 2.5 cm wide.
- Scissors.
- Sterile gloves.

PROCEDURE
Sterile gloves are worn throughout the procedure.
1. Explain the procedure to the patient.
2. Wound toilet will have been performed already (Procedure 42).
3. Using a clean technique, place the non-adherent absorbent dressing, shiny side downwards, on to the wound.
4. Fix the non-adherent absorbent dressing with permeable adhesive tape, ensuring the tape does not encircle the whole limb or trunk by leaving a gap between the ends—this prevents constriction (Figure 43A).
5. If there is likely to be excessive exudate from the wound, extra gauze may be applied over the non-adherent absorbent dressing and taped into position with permeable adhesive tape.

Advice to patients

- Keep the dressing clean and dry.
- If bleeding or pus appear through the dressing, seek further medical attention.
- Follow advice on how long the dressing is to be worn and whether elevation of the limb is necessary.

6. Cover the dressing with cotton conforming bandage around the limb or trunk, and secure the bandage with elastic adhesive tape (Figure 43B).
7. An alternative adhesive dressing can be used (Figure 43C).

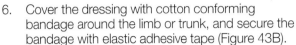
Figure 43A

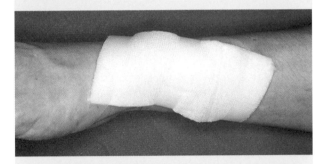
Figure 43B

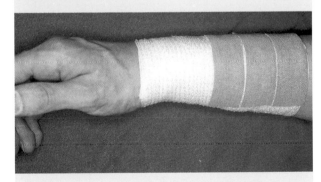
Figure 43C

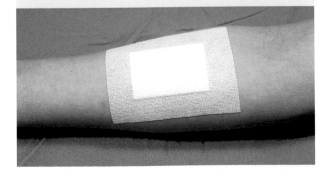

Dressing to a finger or toe

USES
- To protect a broken skin surface on a finger or toe.
- After suturing of a finger or toe.

EQUIPMENT
- Non-adherent absorbent dressing.
- Permeable adhesive tape, 1.25 cm wide.
- Cotton tubular bandage.
- Applicator for cotton tubular bandage.
- Elastic adhesive tape, 2.5 cm wide.
- Scissors.
- Sterile gloves.

PROCEDURE
Sterile gloves are worn throughout the procedure.
1. Explain the procedure to the patient.
2. Wound toilet will have been performed already (Procedure 42) and the wound may have been sutured.
3. Using a clean technique, place the non-adherent absorbent dressing, shiny side downwards, on to the wound.
4. Fix the non-adherent absorbent dressing with permeable adhesive tape, ensuring the tape does not completely encircle the digit (Figure 44A).
5. Select the appropriate width of cotton tubular bandage and cut a length about five times as long as the injured digit. Thread the bandage over the applicator.
6. Pass the applicator over the digit and ease off the end of the bandage; twist the applicator around the base of the digit in order to anchor the bandage.
7. Withdraw the applicator to the end of the digit and then twist the bandage through two complete turns (Figure 44B).
8. Repeat steps 6 and 7.
9. Split the remaining piece of bandage into two and use the two ends to tie the dressing loosely in position at the base of the digit (Figure 44C).
10. Anchor the bandage to the skin at the base of the digit with elastic adhesive tape, snipping at the web space to make it comfortable (Figures 44D and 44E). Ensure that the patient is not allergic to elastic adhesive tape—if the patient is, substitute with a non-allergenic tape.

Figure 44A

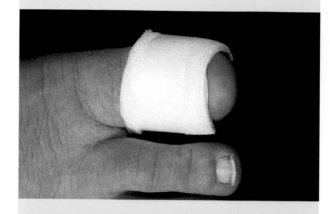

Figure 44B

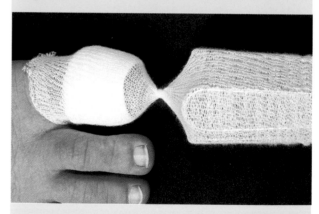

Figure 44C

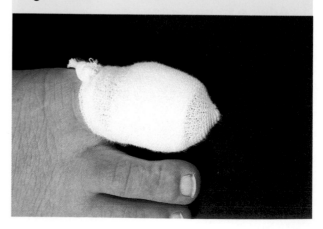

Figure 44D

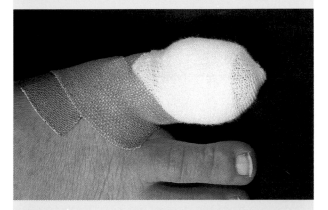

Figure 44E

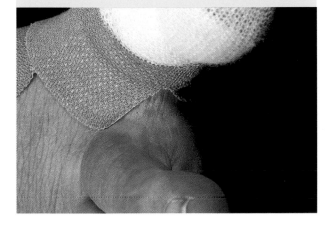

Advice to patients

- Keep the dressing clean and dry.
- If bleeding or pus appear through the dressing, seek further medical attention.
- Follow advice on how long the dressing is to be worn and whether elevation of the limb is necessary.
- The digit can be moved as much as the dressing will allow.

Pressure dressing to the head

USES
- To arrest haemorrhage.
- To prevent the formation of a haematoma.

EQUIPMENT
- Sterile dressing pack, including:
  Tray or receiver.
  Gauze.
  Gloves.
  Towels.
  Gallipot.
- Non-adherent absorbent dressing.
- Absorbent dressing pad.
- Permeable adhesive tape, 1.25 cm wide.
- Two crepe bandages, 10 cm wide.
- Elastic adhesive tape, 2.5 cm wide.
- Scissors.

PROCEDURE
Two people are required for this procedure. Sterile gloves are worn throughout.

1. Wound toilet will have been performed already (Procedure 42) and the wound may have been sutured.
2. Place the non-adherent absorbent dressing, shiny side downwards, on to the wound. Place several layers of gauze over the non-adherent absorbent dressing, to form a pressure pad. Consider adding an absorbent dressing pad if the wound is still bleeding. Tape down with permeable adhesive tape if necessary.
3. Cover the dressing with two layers of the first crepe bandage, applied firmly around the head. Apply the second crepe bandage firmly over the first, in the oppsite direction around the head. Continue with the first bandage, moving from the front of the head to the back of the head and folding the bandage back on itself. Repeat this with the second bandage but covering the head from ear to ear (Figures 45A and 45B). Continue to alternate these

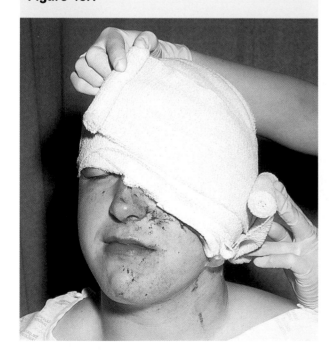

Figure 45A

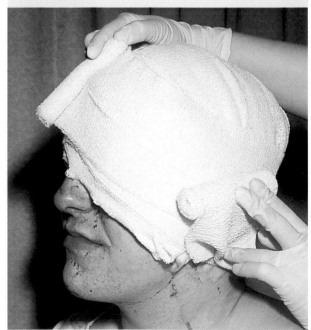

Figure 45B

steps until all of the bandages have been used and the finished dressing covers the head firmly and completely.

4. Secure the ends of the bandages with elastic adhesive tape (Figure 45C).

Advice to patients

- Keep the dressing clean and dry.
- If bleeding or pus appear through the dressing, seek further medical attention.
- Leave the dressing in position for at least 24 hours.
- If indicated, written head injury instructions should be provided.

Figure 45C

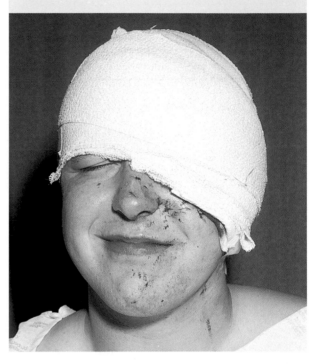

Pressure dressing to a limb

USES
- To arrest haemorrhage.
- To prevent the formation of a haematoma.

EQUIPMENT
- Sterile dressing pack, including:
  Tray or receiver.
  Gauze.
  Gloves.
  Towels.
  Gallipot.
- Non-adherent absorbent dressing.
- Permeable adhesive tape, 1.25 cm wide.
- Crepe bandage.
- Elastic adhesive tape, 2.5 cm wide.
- Scissors.

PROCEDURE
Sterile gloves are worn throughout the procedure.
1. Wound toilet will have been performed already (Procedure 42) and the wound may have been sutured.
2. Place the non-adherent absorbent dressing, shiny side downwards, on to the wound. Place several layers of gauze over the non-adherent absorbent dressing, to form a pressure pad.

Tape down with permeable adhesive tape, ensuring that the tape does not completely encircle the whole limb (Figure 46A).
3. Cover the dressing with a crepe bandage applied firmly around the limb and secure the crepe bandage with elastic adhesive tape (Figure 46B). If the limb is already swollen or is likely to swell, it may be necessary to apply the crepe bandage evenly from joint to joint (e.g. from toes to knee) to avoid constriction.

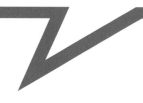

Advice to patients

- Keep the dressing clean and dry.
- If bleeding or pus appear through the dressing, seek further medical attention.
- Leave the dressing in position for at least 24 hours—keep the arm in a sling, or elevate the leg, during this time.

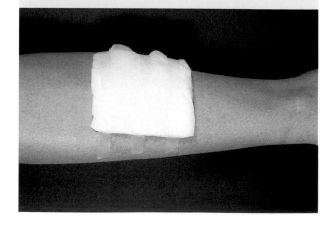

Figure 46A

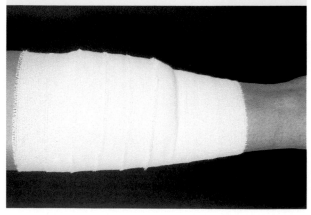

Figure 46B

Pressure dressing to a finger

USE
- To arrest haemorrhage.

EQUIPMENT
- Sterile dressing pack, including:
  Tray or receiver.
  Gauze.
  Gloves.
  Towels.
  Gallipot.
- Non-adherent absorbent dressing.
- Permeable adhesive tape, 1.25 cm wide.
- Cotton tubular bandage.
- Applicator for cotton tubular bandage.
- Elastic adhesive tape, 2.5 cm wide.
- Scissors.

PROCEDURE
Sterile gloves are worn throughout the procedure.
1. Wound toilet will have been performed already (Procedure 42) and the wound may have been sutured. A haemostatic dressing may have been applied.
2. Place the non-adherent absorbent dressing, shiny side downwards, on to the wound. Place several layers of gauze over the non-adherent absorbent dressing, to form a pressure pad. Tape down with permeable adhesive tape, ensuring that the tape does not completely encircle the finger (Figure 47A).
3. Select the appropriate width of cotton tubular bandage and cut a length about 10 times as long as the injured finger. Thread the bandage over the applicator.
4. Pass the applicator over the finger and ease off the end of the bandage; twist the applicator around the base of the finger in order to anchor the bandage.
5. To provide additional pressure, twist the applicator continually while withdrawing it to the end of the finger. At the end of the finger, twist the bandage through two complete turns (Figure 47B).
6. Repeat steps 4 and 5 until the finger has been covered four times.
7. Split the remaining piece of bandage into two and use the two ends to tie the dressing loosely in position at the base of the finger.
8. Anchor the bandage to the skin at the base of the finger with elastic adhesive tape (Figure 47C). Ensure that the patient is not allergic to elastic adhesive tape—if the patient is, substitute with a non-allergenic tape. (An alternative method of securing the dressing, especially useful in children, is illustrated in Figure 47D.)
9. Apply a high sling (Procedure 12).

Figure 47A

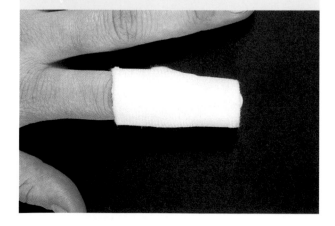

Figure 47B

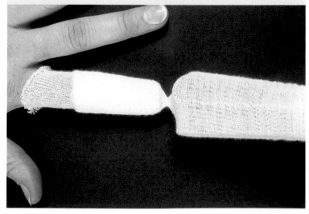

Figure 47C

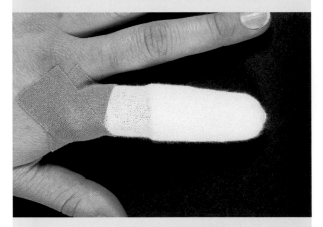

Figure 47D

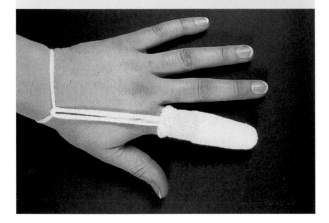

Advice to patients

- Keep the dressing clean and dry.
- If bleeding or pus appear through the dressing, seek further medical attention.
- Leave the dressing in position for at least 24 hours—after this time it is replaced by an ordinary finger dressing (Procedure 44) to allow early mobilization.

48.

Zinc paste and ichthammol bandage

USES
- Lacerations of thin and fragile skin.
- Varicose eczema and leg ulcers.

EQUIPMENT
- Sterile dressing pack, including:
  Tray or receiver.
  Gauze.
  Gloves.
  Towels.
  Gallipot.
- Non-adherent dressing.
- Zinc paste and ichthammol bandage.
- Cotton conforming bandage, 10 cm wide.
- Elastic adhesive tape, 2.5 cm wide.
- Scissors.

PROCEDURE
Sterile gloves are worn throughout the procedure.
1. Wound toilet will have been performed already (Procedure 42) and the wound may have been closed with skin-closure strips and/or sutures.
2. Apply the non-adherent dressing directly over the wound.

3. Beginning about 10 cm below the wound, the zinc paste and ichthammol bandage is applied in a side-to-side fashion, layering it up the limb as necessary. This forms a slab-type cover over the wound. Continue upwards using all the roll of zinc paste and ichthammol bandage and finishing about 10 cm above the wound (Figure 48A). The bandage is therefore not applied around the limb.
4. If there is likely to be excessive exudate from the wound, gauze may be applied over the wound on top of the zinc paste and ichthammol bandage (Figure 48B).
5. For the lower limb, the foot is positioned at a right angle to the lower leg and the cotton conforming bandage is then applied from the base of the toes to just below the knee. This helps optimize the circulation to the wound. Two people may be required for this technique. The cotton conforming bandage is secured with elastic adhesive tape (Figure 48C).
6. For the upper limb, the entire dressing is covered with cotton conforming bandage, secured with elastic adhesive tape.

Figure 48A

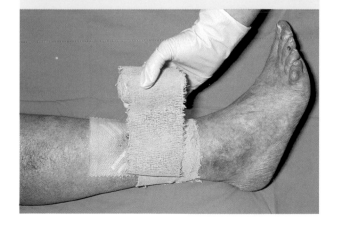

Figure 48B

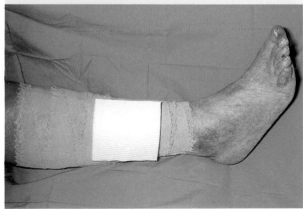

Figure 48C

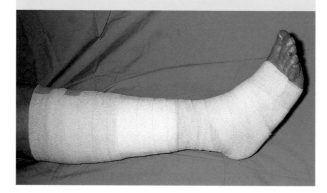

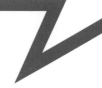

Advice to patients

- Keep the dressing clean and dry.
- If bleeding or exudate appear through the dressing, seek further medical attention.
- Rest the limb and keep it elevated as much as possible.

Burns dressing to a hand, using silver sulphadiazine cream and a burn bag

USE
- To promote healing and prevent infection after a burn or scald of the hand, while encouraging early mobilization.

EQUIPMENT
- Sterile dressing pack, including:
  Tray or receiver.
  Gauze.
  Gloves.
  Towels.
  Gallipot.
- Cleansing solution (e.g. sterile normal saline).
- Sterile needle.
- Sterile scissors.
- Silver sulphadiazine 1% cream.
- Sterile burn bag.
- Cotton conforming bandage, 7.5 cm wide.
- Elastic adhesive tape, 2.5 cm wide.

PROCEDURE
An aseptic technique must be used, and sterile gloves are worn throughout the procedure.
1. Make sure the patient is comfortable, and expose the injured hand and forearm (Figure 49A).
2. A nitrous oxide/oxygen mixture can be used for pain relief (Procedure 87).
3. Clean the area of the burn with a cleansing solution.
4. Either drain the blisters with a sterile needle or remove the tops of the blisters with sterile scissors.
5. Gently cut away any loose skin with sterile scissors.
6. Dry the area completely with gauze.
7. Spread the silver sulphadiazine cream over the area of the burn, using sterile gauze, so that the cream is about 4 mm thick (Figure 49B).

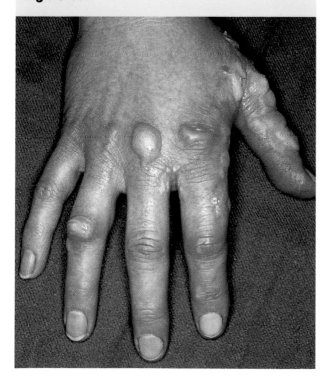

Figure 49A

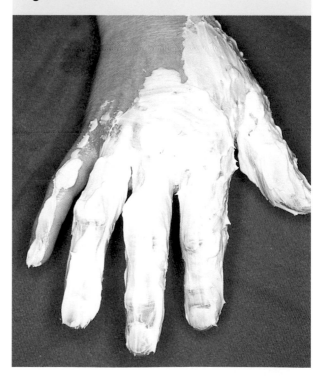

Figure 49B

8. Apply the burn bag over the entire hand and wrist, ensuring that full mobility of the hand is possible inside the bag.
9. Apply several layers of gauze around the wrist to absorb any leakage of exudate, and anchor both the bag and the gauze with cotton conforming bandage around the wrist, securing it with elastic adhesive tape (Figure 49C).
10. Apply a high sling (Procedure 12).

Advice to patients

- Keep the dressing clean and dry.
- If the hand becomes more painful, or inflamed, seek further medical attention.
- Fluid will accumulate in the bag but do not burst the bag as the burn could become infected.
- The silver sulphadiazine cream turns grey after about 24 hours and when it is exposed to daylight, but this is completely harmless.
- Elevate the hand in the high sling.
- Exercise the fingers inside the bag to prevent stiffness.

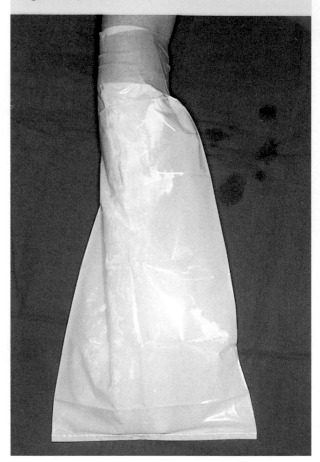

Figure 49C

Suture materials and suturing techniques

SUTURE MATERIALS

Suture materials can be classified as natural or synthetic, absorbable or non-absorbable, and braided or monofilament. Absorbable sutures are usually used when sutures are to be left within the body, e.g. when suturing muscle. Braided sutures are usually easier to tie than monofilament sutures but they tend to harbour bacteria and result in more obvious scarring. Various thicknesses of suture material are available. In the emergency department, the thinnest suture material used is usually 6/0 (used for the face, for example) and the thickest 3/0 or 2/0 (used for the thigh or over a joint, for example).

In the emergency department, interrupted sutures tend to be used more frequently than continuous sutures. This is because only one or two sutures need to be removed if a wound becomes infected, rather than opening the full length of the wound.

Lacerations inside the mouth are often sutured with silk because other materials tend to slip.

Sutures are usually left in place for about six or seven days—however, three or four days may be sufficient in the face, whereas sutures may need to remain in place for more than 10 days over a joint or on the trunk.

SUTURING TECHNIQUES

USES
- To close a wound.

EQUIPMENT
- Sterile suture set, including:
  Scalpel handle.
  Toothed forceps.
  Non-toothed forceps.
  Spencer–Wells forceps.
  Needle holder.
  Sinus forceps.
  Scissors.
  Towels.
  Gauze.
  Tray.
- Cleansing solution (e.g. sterile normal saline).
- Suture material(s).
- Scalpel blade(s).
- Sterile gloves.
- Sterile non-adherent dressing.

PROCEDURE

Requirements for this procedure may include local or general anaesthesia. Good lighting is essential. Sterile gloves are worn throughout. Ensure that the patient is immunized against tetanus.

1. Explain the procedure to the patient. Position the patient lying down, ensuring comfort.
2. Expose the wound—wound toilet will have been performed already (Procedure 42).
3. It may be necessary to excise the edges of the wound if they are dirty or irregular.
4. Use the needle holder to grasp the needle about two-thirds of the distance from the tip (Figure 50A); non-toothed forceps may be used to hold the edges of the wound.
5. Insert the needle into the skin at an angle of 90 degrees. The needle should be inserted far enough from the edge of the wound to prevent the suture from tearing through the skin (Figure 50B).
6. When the tip of the needle is at the base of the wound, release the needle holder and pull the needle out of the wound by its tip with forceps (Figure 50C).
7. The needle is again grasped in the needle holder and inserted into the base of the wound on the opposite side. The needle is pushed up through the skin to the surface and again pulled out, by its tip, with forceps (Figure 50D).

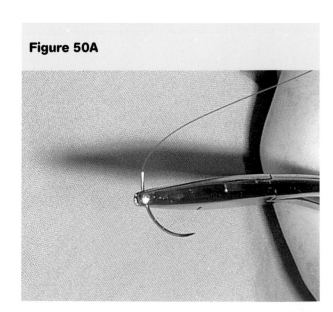

Figure 50A

8. The suture material is then pulled through the wound, leaving a short piece (about 3 cm) at the original point of insertion. The needle is released from the forceps (Figure 50E).
9. The suture material is looped twice round the needle holder. The short end is grasped with the needle holder and pulled through the loops (Figure 50F).
10. The wound edges are brought together with minimal tension, as this first throw of the knot is tied (Figure 50G).
11. A second throw of the knot is formed by looping the suture material around the needle holder and pulling the short end of the material through the loop. If using a monofilament material, additional throws will be required at this stage to prevent slippage.
12. The knots should be laid on one side of the wound and the ends cut to about 5 mm in length to facilitate removal of the sutures at a later date (Figure 50H). When suturing the scalp, the ends of the material are left longer than usual so they can be easily identified at removal.
13. When the entire wound has been sutured, a sterile non-adherent dressing may be applied.

Figure 50C

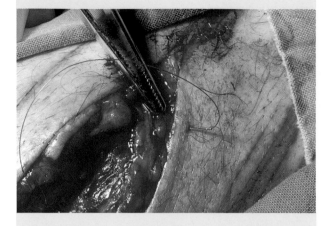

Figure 50D

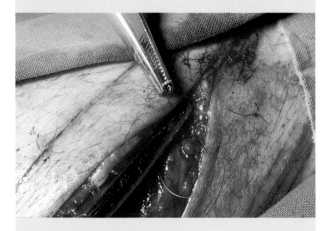

Figure 50B

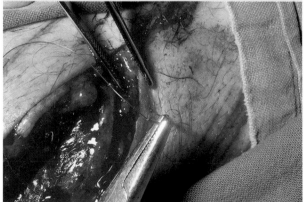

Figure 50E

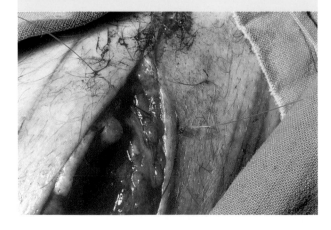

Figure 50F

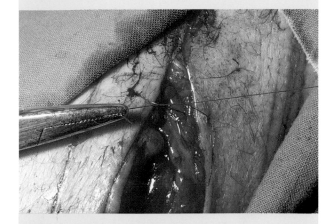

Figure 50G

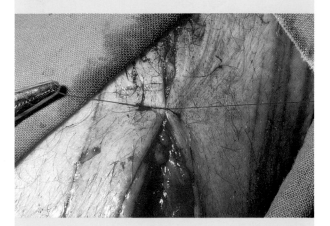

Figure 50H

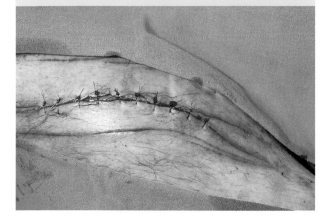

DEEP WOUNDS

In deep wounds, absorbable suture materials are usually used to close the deeper layers of tissue before closing the skin. In this case it is preferable to bury the knots, i.e. put the suture in upside down so that the knot is away from the surface. The needle is introduced at the base of the wound on one side and is brought out halfway up the wound. It is pulled through in the usual manner, inserted at the same level on the opposite side of the wound, and pulled out at the base of the wound. This will place the loose ends of the suture material at the base of the wound so that when they are tied the knots will be buried—this reduces tissue reaction and provides a better cosmetic result.

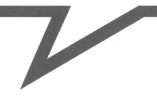

Advice to patients

- Keep the dressing clean and dry.
- If the wound becomes increasingly red or painful or leaks pus, seek further medical attention.
- Exercise, rest, or elevate the injured area as advised.
- Arrange to have the sutures removed as advised.

Skin-closure strips

USE
- To approximate the wound edges in a superficial laceration.

EQUIPMENT
- Sterile dressing pack, including:
  Tray or receiver.
  Gauze.
  Gloves.
  Towels.
  Gallipot.
- Cleansing solution (e.g. sterile normal saline).
- Sterile skin-closure strips.
- Plastic dressing or tincture of benzoin spray.
- Sterile scissors.

PROCEDURE
Good lighting is essential for this procedure. Sterile gloves are worn throughout. Ensure that the patient is immunized against tetanus.
1. Explain the procedure to the patient.
2. Make sure the patient is comfortable, and expose the injured area.
3. Swab the wound until it is clean.
4. Thoroughly dry the area with gauze (Figure 51A).
5. Remove the protective backing from the skin-closure strips.
6. Begin wound closure at the middle of the wound. Apply a skin-closure strip to one side of the wound, pressing it firmly into position; approximate the wound edges and continue the application of the skin-closure strip over the wound and on to the other side of the wound, again pressing it firmly into position (Figure 51B).
7. Position other skin-closure strips in the same way, leaving about a 3 mm gap between the strips, until the wound is closed (Figure 51C).
8. It may be necessary to apply further skin-closure strips parallel to the wound, in order to prevent the edges of the strips from lifting. Plastic dressing or tincture of benzoin spray applied to the area around the wound makes the skin tacky and the strips adhere more easily.
9. Apply a dry dressing (Procedure 43).

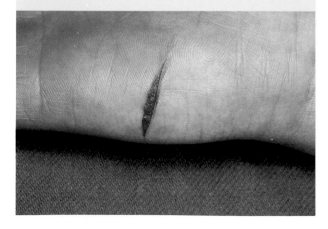

Figure 51A

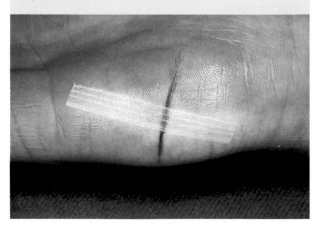

Figure 51B

Figure 51C

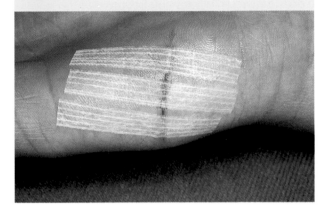

Advice to patients

- Keep the dressing clean and dry.
- If the wound begins to gape, becomes increasingly red or painful, or leaks pus, seek further medical attention.
- Exercise, rest, or elevate the injured area as advised.
- Arrange to have the skin-closure strips removed as advised.

Tissue adhesive

USE

- To close a laceration which is less than about 3 cm in length. Tissue adhesive is particularly useful for lacerations of the scalp, and for children.

CONTRAINDICATIONS

- Tissue adhesive should not be used for:
  - Lacerations which are more than 3 cm in length.
  - Lacerations which are under tension (unless sutures or hair ties have been used to relieve the tension).
  - Lacerations on the eyelids or lips.
  - Deep lacerations.
  - Lacerations with uneven edges.
  - Lacerations which are still bleeding.

EQUIPMENT

- Sterile dressing pack, including:
  Tray or receiver.
  Gauze.
  Gloves.
  Towels.
  Gallipot.
- Tube of tissue adhesive.
- Cleansing solution (e.g. sterile normal saline).
- Sterile scissors.

PROCEDURE

Good lighting is essential for this procedure. Sterile gloves are worn throughout. Ensure that the patient is immunized against tetanus. Two people may be required for this procedure.

1. Explain the procedure to the patient (and to the parents or guardian if necessary).
2. Position the patient lying down, ensuring comfort, and expose the injured area.
3. Clean the laceration with cleansing solution using a modified aseptic technique. Dry the laceration thoroughly (Figure 52A).
4. Snip the tip off the nozzle of the tube of tissue adhesive.
5. Hold the edges of the laceration together—it may be necessary for an assistant to do this.
6. Apply the adhesive in a thin layer, dabbing it along the laceration (Figure 52B). Warn the patient that a slight stinging sensation may be experienced. Within 20 seconds of contact with tissue moisture, the adhesive polymerizes by an exothermic reaction into a firm adhesive bond. Apply tissue adhesive very thinly therefore, to avoid heat damage.
7. Take care not to spill any tissue adhesive and do not allow it to come into contact with your own fingers. Remove any excessive tissue adhesive quickly with a piece of gauze.

Figure 52A

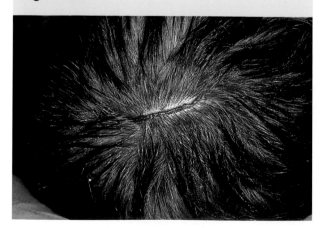

Figure 52B

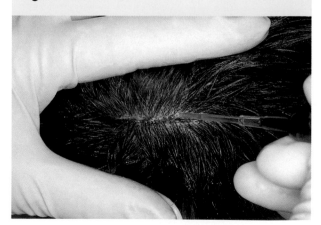

8. Continue to hold the wound edges together for about 30 seconds, while the adhesive dries.
9. Ensure that the laceration is firmly closed (Figure 52C).

Advice to patients

- Leave the wound uncovered (unless the child interferes with it).
- Keep the area as clean and dry as possible but do not wash the area for five days.
- Do not comb hair in the area of the wound or interfere with the eschar.
- After five days, wash the area normally. The tissue adhesive will gradually dissolve or will be removed with the eschar—this may take up to two weeks.
- If the wound begins to bleed, becomes increasingly red or painful, or leaks pus, seek further medical attention.
- The scar may take up to six months to fade.

Figure 52C

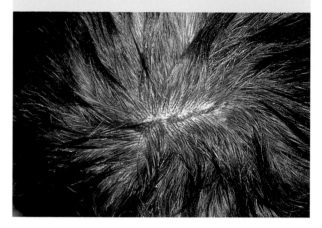

Hair ties

USE
- To close a minor laceration of the scalp. Hair ties are an alternative to suturing or using tissue adhesive—they are particularly useful for children.

EQUIPMENT
- Sterile dressing pack, including:
  Tray or receiver.
  Gauze.
  Gloves.
  Towels.
  Gallipot.
- Cleansing solution (e.g. sterile normal saline).
- Sterile scissors.
- Tube of tissue adhesive.
- Non-heparinized capillary tube.

PROCEDURE
Good lighting is essential for this procedure. Sterile gloves are worn throughout. Ensure that the patient is immunized against tetanus. Two people may be required for this procedure.

1. Explain the procedure to the parents and to the child, simulating the sensation of hair pulling which the patient may experience.
2. Clean the area of the laceration with cleansing solution, ensuring that the laceration can be seen clearly (Figure 53A).
3. Pat the area dry with sterile gauze.
4. Beginning at the centre of the laceration, select four or five strands of hair from either side of the laceration, ensuring that the strands of hair lie in apposition to each other. It may be necessary to trim the hair to a manageable length.
5. Tie the hair strands once across the laceration, to form the beginning of a knot (Figure 53B). Pat the area dry as necessary.
6. The second person draws a little tissue adhesive into the non-heparinized capillary tube and applies a drop of tissue adhesive from the capillary tube on to the centre of the knot (Figure 53C).
7. The knot may then be completed and a further drop of tissue adhesive applied to secure it. Continue this procedure along the laceration (leaving a space between the knots, as in a sutured wound) until the edges of the laceration are opposed (Figure 53D).

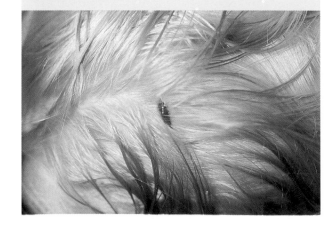

Figure 53A

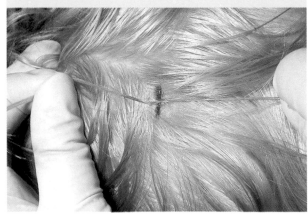

Figure 53B

Figure 53C

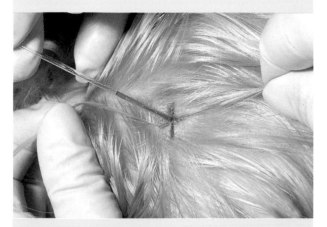

Figure 53D

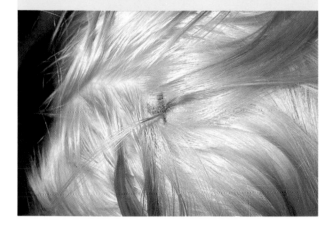

Advice to patients and parents

- Take care when combing the hair to avoid pulling the hair ties.
- Do not wash the hair for five days.
- The hair can be washed after five days, gently rubbing over the knots. If the knots do not untie, they may be trimmed.
- The laceration should be clean after about 10 days.
- If the wound begins to gape, bleed, becomes increasingly red or painful, or leaks pus, seek further medical attention.

Incision and drainage of an abscess

USE
- To release pus from an abscess.

EQUIPMENT
- Sterile suture set, including:
  Scalpel handle.
  Toothed forceps.
  Non-toothed forceps.
  Spencer–Wells forceps.
  Needle holder.
  Sinus forceps.
  Scissors.
  Towels.
  Gauze.
  Tray.
- Scalpel blade(s).
- Volkmann's spoon.
- Ribbon gauze.
- Cleansing solution (e.g. 10% povidone–iodine).
- Topical antiseptic solution (Procedure 56).
- Sterile towels.
- Sterile gloves.
- Bacteriology swab.
- Dry dressing.
- Laboratory request card.

PROCEDURE
General or local anaesthesia is required for this procedure. Sterile gloves are worn throughout.

Local infiltration with 1% plain lignocaine solution may not provide effective anaesthesia in areas of infection because of the acidic pH of the tissues. Furthermore, infiltration may theoretically extend the area of infection.

Ethyl chloride spray may be used to 'freeze' the area before incision but is effective for only a few seconds, if at all. In general, it is not recommended.

For any but the smallest abscesses, a general anaesthetic is recommended.

1. Explain the procedure to the patient. Position the patient lying down, ensuring comfort.
2. Expose the infected area (Figure 54A).
3. Clean the area with cleansing solution and position sterile towels around the area.
4. Incise the lesion and release the pus (Figure 54B).
5. A bacteriology swab is taken (Figure 54C).

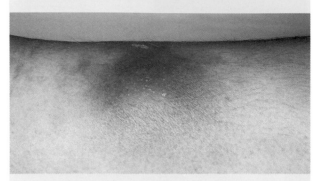

Figure 54A

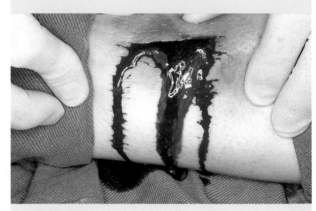

Figure 54B

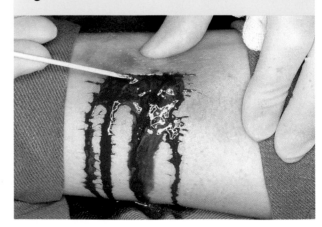

Figure 54C

6. The abscess may need to be curetted with a Volkmann's spoon to break down pockets of infection.
7. The area is irrigated and cleaned (Figure 54D).
8. The ribbon gauze is soaked in topical antiseptic solution and used to pack the wound gently (Figure 54E) (Procedure 55). Packing the wound will aid healing by secondary intention.
9. The wound is covered with gauze and a dry dressing applied (Procedure 43).
10. Label the bacteriology swab, complete the laboratory request card, and send both to the laboratory.
11. Test the patient's urine for glucose.

Figure 54D

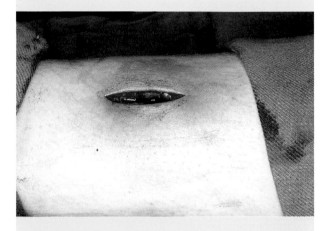

Figure 54E

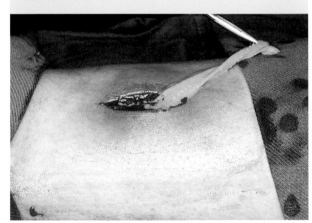

Advice to patients

- Keep the area clean and dry.
- If leakage or bleeding appear through the dressing, seek further medical attention.
- Exercise, rest, or elevate the infected area as advised.
- Arrange further appointments as necessary.
- Take analgesia and antibiotics as prescribed.

Packing of wounds

USE
- To allow an infected wound to heal from its base upwards, by inserting an aseptic wick.

EQUIPMENT
- Sterile dressing pack, including:
  Tray or receiver.
  Gauze.
  Gloves.
  Towels.
  Gallipot.
- Cleansing solution (e.g. sterile normal saline).
- Sterile 10 ml syringe.
- Sterile non-toothed forceps.
- Sterile scissors.
- Topical antiseptic solution (Procedure 56), haemostatic dressing, or petroleum-impregnated ribbon.
- Ribbon gauze; various widths and lengths are available.
- Extra gallipot.

PROCEDURE
Sterile gloves should be worn throughout the procedure.
1. A nitrous oxide/oxygen mixture can be used to relieve pain (Procedure 87).
2. Explain the procedure to the patient.
3. Make sure the patient is comfortable, and expose the area of the wound.
4. Fill the syringe with cleansing solution. Irrigate the wound until it is clean.
5. Thoroughly dry the area with sterile gauze (Figure 55A).
6. Pour some topical antiseptic solution into a gallipot.
7. Using forceps, soak the ribbon gauze in the topical antiseptic solution. If using a haemostatic dressing or petroleum-impregnated ribbon, follow the manufacturer's instructions.
8. Insert one end of the soaked ribbon gauze into the wound and then gently fold it in, completely

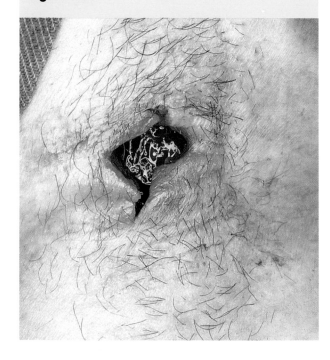

Figure 55A

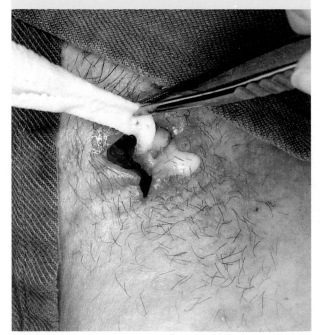

Figure 55B

packing the wound (Figures 55B and 55C). This may cause some discomfort. Cut off any excess ribbon gauze.

9. The ribbon gauze can be packed tightly or loosely.
10. Cover the wound with a suitable dry dressing (Procedure 43).

Advice to patients

- Keep the dressing clean and dry.
- If leakage occurs, seek further medical attention.
- The dressing and pack are likely to require changing in about 24–48 hours.

Figure 55C

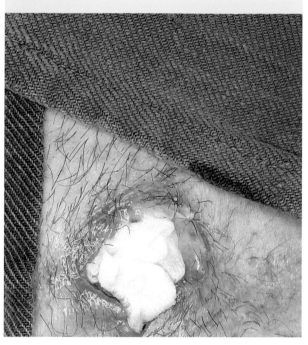

Wound care products, including topical antiseptic solutions

A vast range of wound care products is available and this section describes some of those products which are particularly useful in an emergency department. This is not an exhaustive list and every practitioner has personal preferences. For a comprehensive description of each product, consult the manufacturer's guidelines.

When selecting an appropriate product, consider the following qualities of the ideal wound dressing:
- Protects the wound.
- Impermeable to bacteria.
- Non-adherent.
- Absorbent.
- Comfortable and conformable.
- Non-toxic and non-allergenic.
- Thermally insulating.
- Maintains a high humidity of the wound.
- Allows gaseous exchange of oxygen, carbon dioxide, and water vapour.
- Maintains a constant pH.

LOW ADHERENT DRESSINGS

DRESSING INFORMATION
Many types of low adherent dressings are available (Figure 56A); some consist of a cotton/acrylic viscose absorbent pad, bonded to a perforated film layer, while others comprise single layers of knitted viscose dressings, coated in silicone.

USES
- To cover sutured wounds, superficial grazes, and superficial burns.
- As a low adherent layer between the wound and an antiseptic/antibacterial dressing.
- On infected wounds.

HINTS ON APPLICATION AND ADVICE TO PATIENTS
- Ensure that the correct size of low adherent dressing is selected to avoid a bulky dressing which may impair movement, e.g. in injuries of the fingers where mobilization is important.
- Additional layers of gauze may be required to absorb exudate.
- In a wound that is exuding heavily, advise an early review for a change of dressing if exudate leaks through the dressing.

- For simple wounds or for sutured wounds with minimal exudate, the dressing (if kept dry) can remain in place until the wound has healed or the sutures require removal.

TULLE DRESSINGS

DRESSING INFORMATION
Tulle dressings (Figure 56B) are sheets of gauze impregnated with paraffin and/or antiseptics or other agents (e.g. chlorhexidine); they are available in various sizes.

Figure 56A

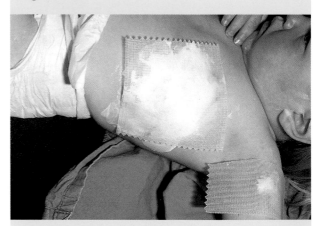

Figure 56B

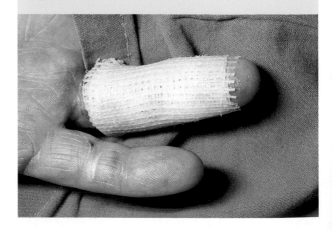

USES

- To cover wounds with low or moderate exudate, e.g. superficial burns and grazes.
- For fingertip injuries, and for infected wounds.

HINTS ON APPLICATION AND ADVICE TO PATIENTS

- Several layers of tulle dressing should be applied to minimize adherence to the surface of the wound.
- Frequent changes of dressing are advisable.
- An additional layer of gauze is required over the tulle dressing to absorb exudate.
- An antibacterial cream may be used in conjunction with tulle dressing.
- Advise the patient to keep the dressing dry and to return if there is leakage through the dressing.
- Allergic reactions to tulle dressings impregnated with antiseptics are not uncommon in patients with leg ulcers; advise the patient to return if the wound becomes irritable or more painful.

POLYSACCHARIDE DRESSINGS

DRESSING INFORMATION

Some polysaccharide dressings (Figure 56C) contain cadexomer iodine, which absorbs pus and exudate and reduces bacterial numbers at the surface of the wound. Polysaccharide dressings are available as granules, paste, or beads, or impregnated in gauze pads or ointment—they should be used with particular

Figure 56C

care in patients with thyroid disorders, because of the potential systemic absorption of iodine, and in patients who are known to be sensitive to iodine. Polysaccharide dressings should not be used in pregnant or lactating patients, or in very young children. When used over a large surface area, be aware of potential systemic absorption of iodine.

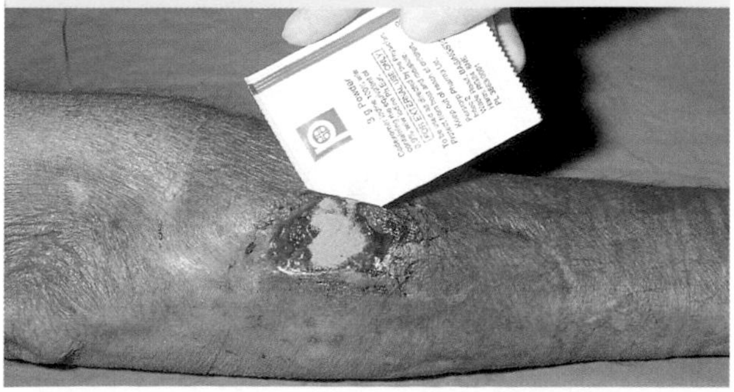

USES

- To cleanse and debride sloughy or necrotic wounds, e.g. leg ulcers and infected traumatic wounds.
- Can be used for cavities and infected wounds.

HINTS ON APPLICATION AND ADVICE TO PATIENTS

- A gauze and/or a low adherent dressing layer will be required over the polysaccharide dressing.
- To ensure that the granules or beads remain inside a cavity, sterile lubricating jelly may be applied to the layer of gauze, or around the perimeter of the wound.
- A change of dressing is usually required every three to five days.
- Ensure that any remaining gel is gently irrigated away with sterile water or sterile normal saline.
- Warn the patient that a little discomfort may be experienced initially after application of the dressing, and advise an early return if this discomfort continues.
- The dressing must be kept dry.

ALGINATES

DRESSING INFORMATION

Alginates consist of a non-woven calcium sodium alginate fibre, in the form of sheets, ribbons, or wicks. The fibres absorb exudate from the wound and the dressing becomes a gel, providing a moist environment for healing.

USES

- To cover wounds which are likely to produce moderate or heavy exudate.
- As a haemostatic agent in certain areas of tissue loss, e.g. fingertip injuries (Figures 56D and 56E), or pre-tibial lacerations with skin loss.

- To pack an incised abscess (as an alternative to ribbon gauze). (Procedures 54 and 55.)
- For infected wounds.

HINTS ON APPLICATION AND ADVICE TO PATIENTS

- Alginates can be used under vapour-permeable films or under layers of gauze; they should be trimmed to the size of the wound and applied to the moist areas.
- Removal of the dressing may be aided by irrigating the area gently with warmed saline solution; because the alginate is biodegradable, any remaining dressing can be left in place.
- An alginate dressing can remain undisturbed for up to seven days, depending upon the amount of exudate.
- Advise the patient to keep the dressing dry.

HYDROGELS

DRESSING INFORMATION

Hydrogel dressings are available in the form of a sheet or ready-mixed gel containing modified carboxymethyl cellulose polymer (Figures 56F, 56G, and 56H).

USES

- To provide a moist environment, facilitating granulation and epithelialization in dermal or superficial burns, and at donor sites.
- The gel can be squeezed into cavities (e.g. leg ulcers, incised abscesses) to debride and deslough these deeper wounds.
- Sheets or gel may be used in areas of localized infection.

HINTS ON APPLICATION AND ADVICE TO PATIENTS

- A gauze and/or a low adherent dressing layer will be required over the ready-mixed gel dressing.
- Hydrogel sheets may remain in place for up to seven days.
- A cavity dressing may require more frequent changes and its removal is aided by gently irrigating the wound with warmed normal saline solution.
- Advise the patient to keep the dressing dry and to return if leakage occurs.

Figure 56D

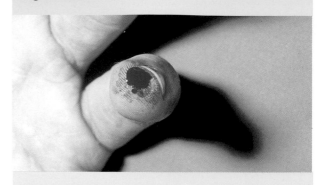

Figure 56E

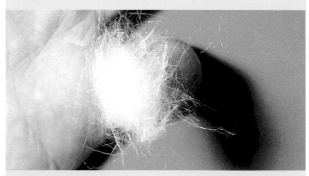

Figure 56F

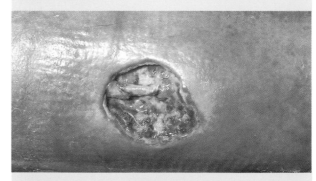

Figure 56G

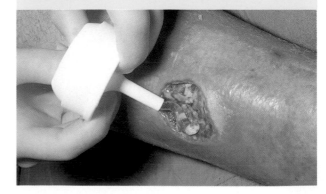

MEDICATED VISCOSE DRESSINGS

DRESSING INFORMATION
Medicated viscose dressings are knitted fabric sheets impregnated with 10% povidone-iodine ointment, which possesses antibacterial properties (Figure 56I). The dressings should be used with particular care in patients with thyroid disorders, because of the potential systemic absorption of iodine, and in patients who are known to be sensitive to iodine. These dressings should not be used in pregnant or lactating patients, or in very young children. When used over a large surface area, be aware of potential systemic absorption of iodine.

USES
* As a prophylactic agent to reduce the risk of infection or to treat infected wounds, e.g. superficial burns, dog bites, infected leg ulcers, and grazes.

HINTS ON APPLICATION AND ADVICE TO PATIENTS
* Medicated viscose dressings may adhere to the surface of the wound and it is therefore advisable to apply them over a low adherent dressing.
* Up to four layers of medicated viscose dressings may be applied, and an additional layer of gauze is necessary to absorb any exudate.
* The dressing may be left in place for up to five days, although antibacterial activity is probably ineffective after 48 hours.
* Warn the patient that the dressing may sting slightly initially but to return if this continues.
* Advise the patient to keep the dressing dry and to return if leakage occurs.

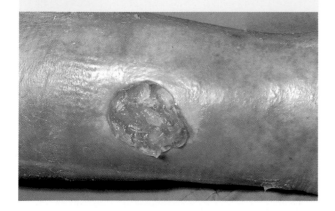

Figure 56H

VAPOUR-PERMEABLE FILMS

DRESSING INFORMATION
Vapour-permeable films consist of a transparent polyurethane film coated with a synthetic adhesive (Figure 56J). The dressings are available in sheets of various sizes; these are conformable and resistant to tearing. Take particular care in areas which are potentially or actually infected, as the occlusive nature of the dressing provides an ideal environment for anaerobic bacteria.

USES
* To provide an occlusive, moist, warm environment, which aids granulation and epithelialization; therefore useful for superficial burns and abrasions.
* Their occlusive properties provide a good analgesic effect by covering exposed nerve endings.
* As a dressing at the site of insertion of an intravenous cannula.

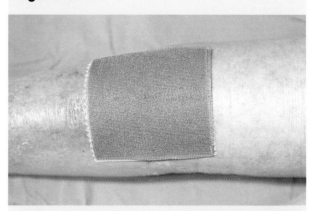

Figure 56I

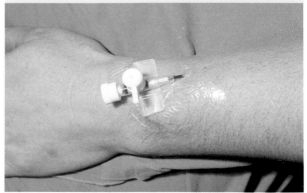

Figure 56J

HINTS ON APPLICATION AND ADVICE TO PATIENTS

- The semi-permeable membrane of vapour-permeable films allows excess exudate to evaporate, thus preventing maceration of the wound. However, a more absorbent dressing may be required in a wound with moderate or heavy exudate.
- Application of these dressings may be difficult over a large area or in a non-cooperative patient such as a child; two people may be required to apply the dressings in these circumstances.
- The dressing permits observation and assessment of the wound. The patient may request that a light conforming bandage is applied over the dressing for aesthetic reasons.
- Removal of the dressing may cause discomfort but this can be minimized by lifting the edge of the dressing and pulling it horizontally before lifting upwards.
- The dressing is waterproof and so the patient can wash and bathe while it is in place.
- The dressing can be left on for up to seven days.
- Advise the patient to return early if leakage occurs.

HYDROCOLLOID DRESSINGS

DRESSING INFORMATION

Hydrocolloid dressings consist of a mixture of gelatins, pectins, and elastomers. They are available as wafer-type squares of various sizes and thicknesses; they are also available as powders, pastes, and granules. When the hydrocolloid comes into contact with secretions from the wound, it dissolves into a gel, providing an ideal environment for moist wound healing. Hydrocolloid dressings are occlusive and should therefore be avoided in areas of potential infection as they provide an ideal environment for anaerobic bacteria.

USES

- To cover superficial and dermal layer burns, leg ulcers, and any granulating or epithelializing wound (Figures 56K and 56L).
- To rehydrate eschars and promote autolysis on necrotic wounds
- For fingertip injuries.

HINTS ON APPLICATION AND ADVICE TO PATIENTS

- When applying a hydrocolloid wafer, leave a 5 cm border around the wound; in leg injuries it is advisable to leave a larger border below the wound to retain any exudate gravitating downwards from the wound.
- Warn the patient that the gel which forms has an unpleasant smell.
- The thinner wafers can be cut into a 'T' shape to dress a fingertip from which tissue has been avulsed.

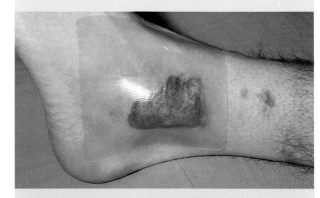

Figure 56L

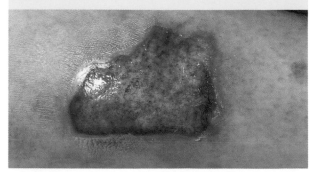

Figure 56K

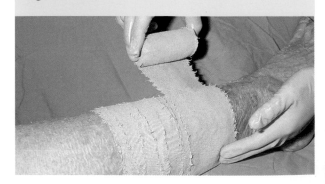

Figure 56M

* A hydrocolloid dressing can be left in place for up to five days, provided there is no leakage.
* The dressing is waterproof and so the patient can wash and bathe while it is in place.

PASTE BANDAGES

DRESSING INFORMATION

Paste bandages consist of open-weave cotton bandages, impregnated with antibacterial paste such as zinc oxide and ichthammol (Figure 56M, Procedure 48).

USES

* To cover leg ulcers, pre-tibial lacerations (which may have been treated with skin-closure strips), torn skin, and superficially avulsed tissues.
* On fragile skin, e.g. frail, elderly patients and patients on long-term steroid therapy.
* They can be used on infected wounds.

HINTS ON APPLICATION AND ADVICE TO PATIENTS

* A low adherent dressing may be placed directly over a wound before the application of a paste bandage.
* An absorbent gauze pad may be required over the paste bandage to absorb any exudate; this should be held in position with a cotton conforming bandage.
* Apply the paste bandage by pleating or folding the layers across the wound or along the limb: the paste bandage has no elastic properties and could act as a tourniquet if it was wrapped around the limb.
* A patient with venous insufficiency may require a graduated compression bandage along the length of the leg, from toes to knee.
* The paste bandage retains moisture and can therefore be left in place for up to two weeks.
* The patient must keep the dressing dry and should return early if leakage occurs.

VAPOUR-PERMEABLE FILMS CONTAINING SILVER

DRESSING INFORMATION

Vapour-permeable films consist of a semi-permeable polyurethane film with a self-adhesive surface. The polyurethane film contains a formulation of silver which is released in a controlled amount (Figure 56N). Because of its occlusive nature, the film dressing creates a moist healing environment, and the constant slow release of silver ions provides a continuous antibacterial effect.

USES

* To encourage epithelialization in a wound, e.g. superficial and dermal layer burns, abrasions, and leg ulcers.
* In areas of localized infection.

HINTS ON APPLICATION AND ADVICE TO PATIENTS

* As the vapour-permeable film has minimal absorbent properties, an alginate dressing may be placed over an exuding or bleeding wound, and the film layer placed over the top of the alginate dressing.
* The vapour-permeable film may be difficult to apply and two people may be required.
* A border (about 3–5 cm) should be left around the wound.
* The dressing is designed to be left in place for up to seven days, provided there is no leakage; however, by this time the antibacterial properties of the dressing will be minimal.
* The dressing is waterproof and the patient can wash and bathe.

CLING FILM

Cling film is useful as a first aid measure for a patient who has sustained a burn (Figure 56O). As cling film is occlusive it provides analgesic benefits, and the burn can also be reassessed without being disturbed. Cling film is useful before transportation of a patient to a burns unit; it reduces the risk of hypothermia, which is a recognized complication of

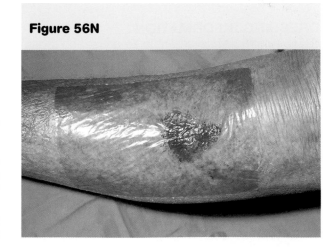

Figure 56N

applying saline-soaked towels. Cling film is laid over the burn in strips, to prevent a tourniquet-type effect. If a burn is large, two people will be required to apply the cling film.

CLEANSING SOLUTIONS

The most usual cleansing solution used in the emergency department is **sterile normal saline** (0.9% sodium chloride solution). It causes minimal tissue damage and is most effective if warmed and gently irrigated into the wound.

If a strict aseptic technique is required (such as for aspiration of a knee or intraosseous infusion), it may be advisable to use **10% povidone-iodine solution**, which is also useful for particularly dirty wounds and compound fractures (Figure 56P).

Hydrogen peroxide solution is a colourless antiseptic liquid. It is most often used as a 6% solution in water which releases 20 times its own volume of oxygen—this strength is also known as 20-volume strength. Solutions stronger than 6% must be diluted before use. Hydrogen peroxide is useful for cleaning infected wounds, bites, and ulcers. It bubbles when it comes into contact with tissues, and oxygen is released (Figure 56Q); this is particularly advantageous for wounds containing tiny particles of dirt. It helps to separate discharges and is effective against both aerobic and anaerobic organisms. Following irrigation with hydrogen peroxide, the wound should be thoroughly irrigated with sterile normal saline before further treatment. Hydrogen peroxide potentiates povidone-iodine by increasing the release of available iodine. It bleaches fabrics.

TOPICAL ANTISEPTIC SOLUTIONS

SILVER SULPHADIAZINE CREAM

DRESSING INFORMATION
Silver sulphadiazine cream is an antiseptic cream containing 1% silver sulphadiazine. It is effective against both Gram-positive and Gram-negative bacteria but not against spores. It is particularly effective against *Pseudomonas*. Silver sulphadiazine cream occasionally causes hypersensitivity and leucopenia. It is contraindicated in pregnancy and during lactation, in infants under three months old, and in patients who are sensitive to sulphonamides. It should be used with caution if there is impaired function of the kidneys or liver. If the cream is used on full-thickness burns, it may mask the appearance of the burn so that subsequent assessment of the burn is difficult.

USES
- For burns (Figure 56R), wounds, infected leg ulcers, and skin graft donor sites.
- Its occlusive properties provide a considerable analgesic effect, particularly in burns.
- Reduces the risk of infection, for example in burns, leg ulcers, and fingertip injuries.
- Following crushing injuries or injuries which have resulted in the loss of tissue.

Figure 56O

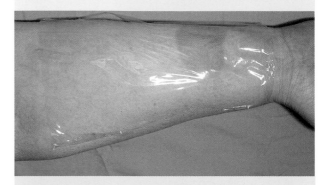

Figure 56P

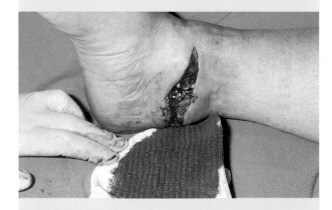

Figure 56Q

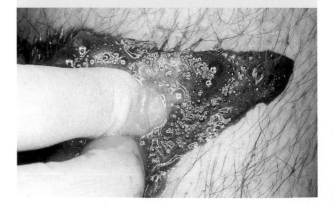

HINTS ON APPLICATION AND ADVICE TO PATIENTS

- Apply the silver sulphadiazine cream by dabbing it on to the wound in a layer which is approximately 4 mm thick.
- Apply a low adherent dressing over the cream and then apply gauze and cotton conforming bandage.
- A sterile burn bag can be used to cover a hand that has had silver sulphadiazine cream applied to a burn (Procedure 49).
- If the area of injury is relatively flat, a vapour-permeable film dressing can be applied over the silver sulphadiazine cream.
- For an injury of the fingertip, silver sulphadiazine cream can be applied and the injured finger can then be covered with the finger of a sterile glove.
- The patient should be warned that the silver sulphadiazine cream turns grey after about 24 hours and when it is exposed to daylight, but this is completely harmless. Avoid using it on the face.
- The antibacterial properties of the cream are greatly reduced after about 48 hours and so the dressing is usually changed every couple of days.
- The patient must keep the dressing dry and must return early if there is any leakage through the dressing.

POVIDONE-IODINE OINTMENT

Povidone-iodine ointment is an antiseptic agent containing 10% povidone-iodine. It is useful for the management of burns (Figure 56S) and wounds, and is effective against all bacterial species, and against spores, fungi, and viruses. Povidone-iodine should be used with caution in pregnant and lactating patients, and in patients with renal impairment. Its use may interfere with thyroid function tests. Sensitivity can occur. It can stain clothes.

PROFLAVINE CREAM

Proflavine cream is a bright yellow antiseptic agent. It can be used for packing wounds (Figure 56T, Procedure 55) and for infected ulcers. Proflavine cream is effective against both Gram-positive and Gram-negative bacteria but not against spores. It is not inactivated by body fluids or pus. It is non-irritating and non-toxic but it stains clothes. Wounds packed with proflavine cream should be reviewed at least every 48 hours.

Figure 56R

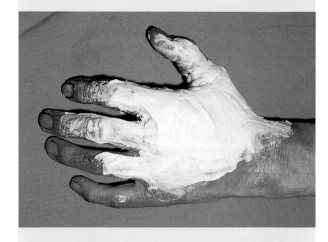

Figure 56S

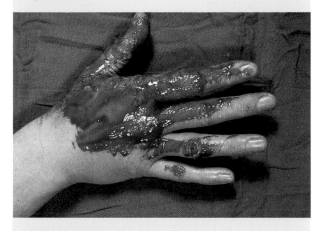

Figure 56T

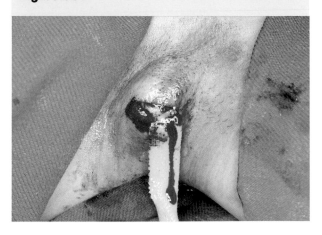

Maintenance of the airway

USE
- To maintain the airway, particularly in the unconscious patient. **Following trauma, maintenance of the airway must be achieved without hyperextension of the cervical spine.**

EQUIPMENT
- Magill's forceps.
- Suction apparatus, including a wide-bore rigid (Yankauer) catheter and smaller flexible catheters.

PROCEDURES
Muscular control of the tongue is lost in unconscious patients, and the following manoeuvres may be required to maintain the airway.
1. Look, listen, and feel for breathing.
2. If the airway is unsatisfactory, open the patient's mouth and remove any obvious obstructions, e.g. loose teeth or broken or displaced dentures. A finger sweep or Magill's forceps can be used to clear the mouth.
3. Secretions and vomitus may be removed by gentle suction.

Chin lift
4. Place one of your hands on the patient's forehead so as to stabilize the head and neck.
5. Simultaneously, place two fingers of your other hand under the tip of the mandible and lift the chin (Figure 57A).

Jaw thrust
4. Hold the patient's mouth slightly open by downwards displacement of the chin with your thumbs.
5. Place your fingers behind the angles of the mandible and apply steady upwards and forwards pressure in order to lift the jaw forwards (Figure 57B).

Figure 57A

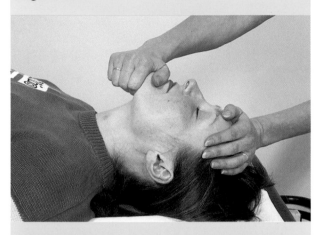

Figure 57B

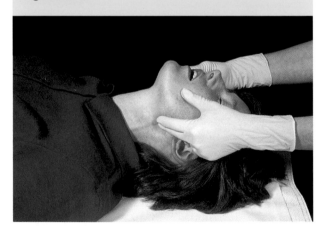

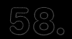

Mouth-to-mouth ventilation

USE
- To ventilate an apnoeic patient. To diagnose apnoea, look for chest movements, listen for breath sounds at the mouth, and feel for air with your cheek.

EQUIPMENT
No special equipment is required for mouth-to-mouth ventilation. However, certain interpositional airway devices are available for the protection and aesthetic convenience of the practitioner.

PROCEDURE
1. Place the patient in a supine position, open the airway, and remove any obvious obstructions from the mouth, e.g. loose dentures.
2. Ensure the head is tilted backwards.
3. Pinch the patient's nostrils with your index finger and thumb, to occlude the nose.
4. Support the chin with your other hand and allow the mouth to open slightly.
5. Take a deep breath and seal your lips around the patient's mouth.
6. Blow steadily into the patient's mouth and watch the chest rise (Figure 58)—allow about two seconds for the full inflation. If the chest does not rise, check that the airway is clear, that the head is tilted back sufficiently, and that you have made a good seal with your lips.
7. Maintaining head tilt and chin lift, take your mouth away from the patient at the end of inspiration to allow passive expiration by the patient. Watch the chest fall.
8. Continue at a rate of about 10 breaths per minute.
9. Check the pulse after every 10 breaths, instituting full cardiopulmonary resuscitation if the pulse disappears.

Figure 58

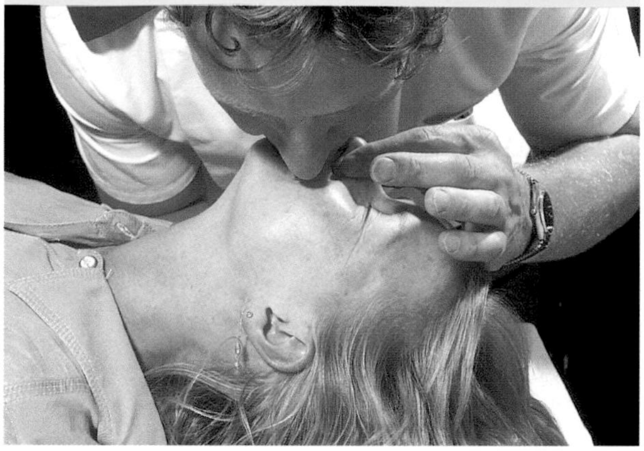

Mouth-to-nose ventilation

USE
- To ventilate an apnoeic patient. Mouth-to-nose ventilation may be preferable to mouth-to-mouth ventilation if the latter is technically difficult, e.g. because of unusual or absent dentition. Mouth-to-nose ventilation can also be used: if an obstruction in the mouth cannot be relieved; during recovery of a patient in water when one hand is needed to support the body so cannot be used to close the nose; by a child whose mouth may not be large enough to form a seal with an adult's mouth.

EQUIPMENT
No special equipment is required for mouth-to-nose ventilation.

PROCEDURE
1. Place the patient in a supine position and remove any obvious obstructions from the airway.
2. Tilt the patient's head back, using your other hand to support the chin and to keep the mouth closed.
3. Take a deep breath and seal your lips around the patient's nose.
4. Blow steadily into the patient's nose and watch the chest rise (Figure 59)—allow about two seconds for the full inflation.
5. Assist passive expiration by opening the patient's mouth. Watch the chest fall.
6. Continue at a rate of about 10 breaths per minute.
7. Check the pulse after every 10 breaths, instituting full cardiopulmonary resuscitation if the pulse disappears.

Figure 59

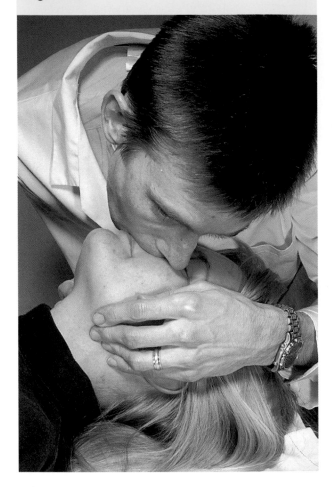

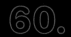

Insertion of an oropharyngeal or nasopharyngeal airway

USE
- To maintain the airway, usually in an unconscious patient.

EQUIPMENT
- Oropharyngeal (Guedel) airways: usually size 2, 3, or 4 for adults of small, medium, or large build respectively.
- Nasopharyngeal airways: usually sizes 6–8 mm (internal diameter) for adults.
- Safety pin.
- Water-soluble lubricant.
- Suction apparatus.

PROCEDURES
Oropharyngeal airway
1. Select an oropharyngeal airway which corresponds in length to the distance from the corner of the patient's mouth to the angle of the jaw (Figure 60A).
2. Open the patient's mouth and remove any foreign material.
3. Insert the oropharyngeal airway with the tip facing towards the roof of the mouth (Figure 60B). As the oropharyngeal airway passes the back of the tongue, rotate it through 180 degrees.
4. If the patient coughs or retches, remove the oropharyngeal airway to avoid stimulating vomiting or severe laryngospasm.
5. The flange of the oropharyngeal airway will now rest against the outside of the patient's lips. Ensure that the lips are clear of the teeth to avoid damage (Figure 60C).
6. After insertion of the oropharyngeal airway, look, listen, and feel for breathing.

Nasopharyngeal airway
A nasopharyngeal airway can be used in conscious patients (especially in patients with clenched jaws or trismus) and in unconscious patients. It is contraindicated if the patient has a suspected or confirmed fracture of the base of the skull.
1. Measure the nasopharyngeal airway from the tip of the patient's nose to the earlobe, to determine the correct length (Figure 60D). Nasopharyngeal airways are sized in millimetres according to their internal diameter, the length increasing with the diameter. Sizes used in adults are usually

Figure 60A

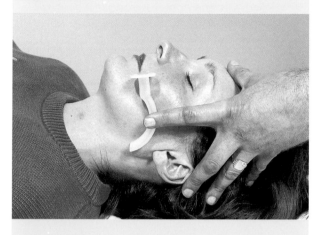

Figure 60B

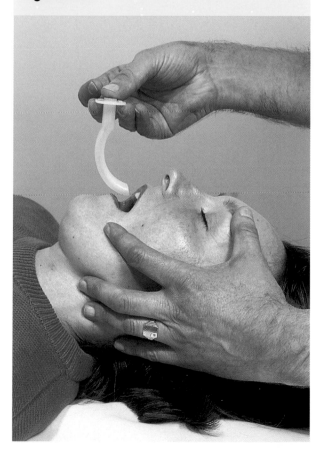

6–8 mm (about the same diameter as the patient's little finger). Use the largest size that will fit into the patient's nostril.

2. Check the patency of the patient's nostril.
3. Insert a safety pin through the flange of the nasopharyngeal airway to prevent it from being inhaled.
4. Lubricate the nasopharyngeal airway.
5. Insert the nasopharyngeal airway, bevel-end leading, into the nostril. Introduce it directly backwards along the floor of the nose with a clockwise–anti-clockwise twisting action.
6. Continue to direct the airway posteriorly until the flange (with the safety pin through it) rests against the nostril: the tip of the airway will now lie in the pharynx (Figure 60E).
7. If resistance is encountered, remove the airway and try the other nostril.
8. Suction must be available, in case the procedure results in an epistaxis.
9. After insertion of the nasopharyngeal airway, look, listen, and feel for breathing.

Figure 60C

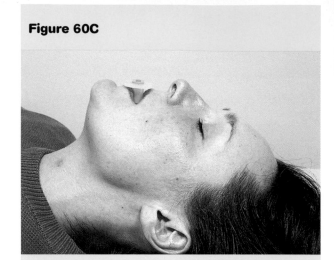

Figure 60D

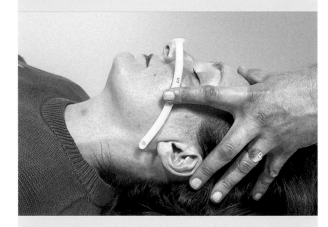

Figure 60E

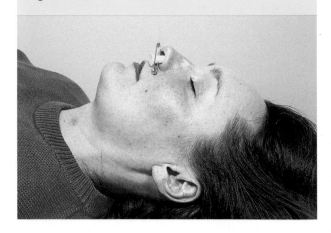

Manual ventilation

USE
- To allow high concentrations of oxygen to be delivered to the patient. Manual ventilation requires training and practice. A self-inflating bag with a one-way valve is most commonly used, with either a facemask or an endotracheal tube.

EQUIPMENT
- Oropharyngeal (Guedel) airway.
- Self-inflating bag with attached facemask of an appropriate size.
- Oxygen reservoir bag attached to the self-inflating bag.
- Oxygen supply with attached tubing.
- Gloves.

PROCEDURE
1. Place the patient in a supine position. Wear gloves.
2. Open the patient's airway and insert an oropharyngeal airway (Procedure 60).
3. Apply a facemask of appropriate size over the patient's nose and mouth. Hold the facemask in position by curling the thumb and index finger of one hand around the connection of the facemask with the self-inflating bag.
4. Apply upwards pressure on the patient's chin, using your little and ring fingers to provide a jaw thrust manoeuvre (Figure 61A).
5. Apply enough pressure to ensure an airtight seal between the facemask and the patient's face.
6. Use your other hand to squeeze the self-inflating bag, with the oxygen and reservoir bag attached to it. Ensure that the reservoir bag remains fully inflated during ventilation (Figure 61B). Oxygen delivery should be set at a rate of 15 litres per minute.
7. Watch the chest rise.
8. Release the self-inflating bag to allow passive expiration by the patient. Watch the chest fall.

Figure 61A

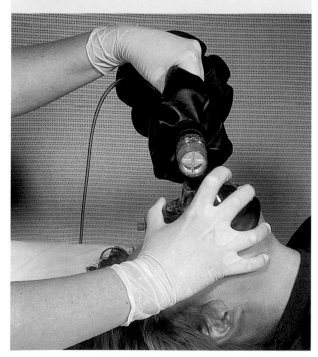

Figure 61B

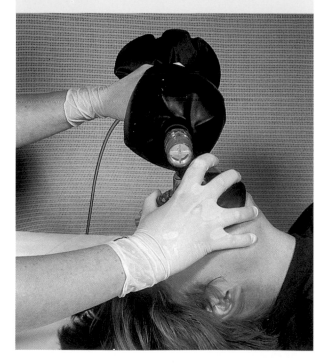

9. Continue at a rate of about 12–15 breaths per minute.
10. The technique is more efficient if two people are involved. One person holds the facemask in position, using both hands to ensure an airtight seal and to maintain the jaw thrust manoeuvre. The assistant squeezes and releases the self-inflating bag (Figure 61C).
11. Endotracheal intubation can overcome the difficulties of using a facemask. It eliminates leaks and ensures that oxygen is delivered to the lungs and not to the stomach.

Figure 61C

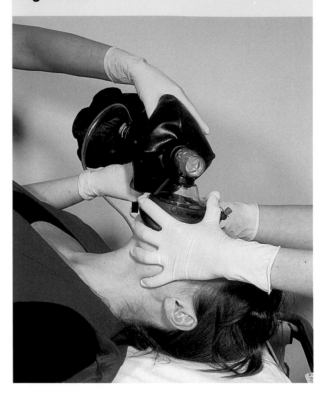

Relief of choking

USE
- To clear the airway blocked by a foreign body (usually food).

EQUIPMENT
No special equipment is required to relieve choking.

PROCEDURE IN AN ADULT
1. If the patient is conscious and breathing, encourage him or her to continue coughing but do nothing else.
2. If obstruction is complete and the patient shows signs of exhaustion or becomes cyanosed but is still conscious, stand to the side and slightly behind; support the chest with one hand and lean the patient well forwards; deliver up to five sharp blows to the patient's back between the scapulae with the heel of your free hand.
3. If this fails to clear the obstruction, try abdominal thrusts (Heimlich's manoeuvre). Stand behind the patient, put both your arms around the upper abdomen, clench your fist and grasp it with your other hand; pull sharply inwards and upwards in order to produce a sudden expulsion of air, together with the foreign body, from the airway (Figure 62A).
4. If still unsuccessful, alternate five back blows with five abdominal thrusts.
5. If the patient is unconscious, try to remove the foreign body with finger sweeps. If unsuccessful, give a series of abdominal thrusts with the patient lying supine on the floor. Alternatively, chest thrusts similar to the technique of chest compressions during cardiac arrest may be successful.

PROCEDURE IN A CHILD
1. Lay the child, face down, across your lap. Give five sharp back blows between the shoulders.
2. If this fails, stand behind the child and pass your arms around the body. Place your clenched fist against the child's upper abdomen, place your other hand over the fist, and thrust both hands sharply upwards into the abdomen (Figure 62B). Repeat this 10 times, unless the obstruction is relieved before then. This procedure may be more effective if the child is able to stand on a box or chair.

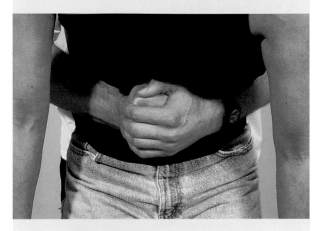

Figure 62A

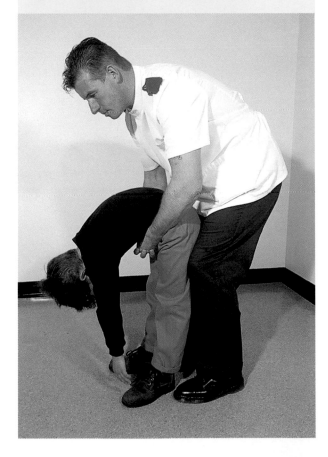

Figure 62B

3. If the child is supine, kneel at his or her feet, or astride the child. Place the heel of your hand against the upper abdomen. Place your other hand on top of the first and thrust both hands sharply upwards into the abdomen, taking care to direct the thrust in the midline. Repeat this 10 times unless the obstruction is relieved before then.

PROCEDURE IN A BABY

1. Place the baby along your forearm with the face and head down, and support the head and shoulders with your hand.
2. Give five sharp slaps on the baby's back with the heel of your free hand (Figure 62C).
3. If this fails to relieve the obstruction, turn the baby over to lie along your thigh, still with the head down. Give five sharp thrusts to the lower chest, using two fingers only.
4. Do not use abdominal thrusts in babies as these may cause intra-abdominal injury.

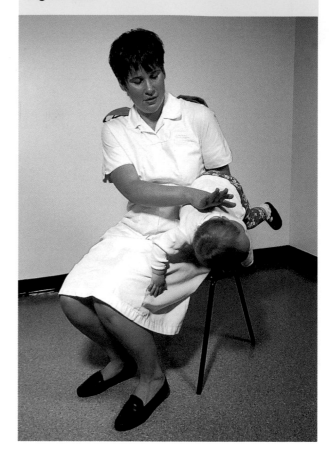

Figure 62C

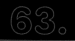

Endotracheal intubation

USE
In an unconscious patient:
* To provide and maintain an airway.
* To prevent aspiration of gastric contents.

EQUIPMENT
* Cuffed endotracheal tube of appropriate size, fitted with a 15 mm connector:
  * Male adults usually require an endotracheal tube of internal diameter 8–9 mm, cut to a length of 23–26 cm.
  * Female adults usually require an endotracheal tube of internal diameter 7–8 mm, cut to a length of 20–22 cm.
  * Children require endotracheal tubes of various sizes (Procedure 69).
* Water-soluble lubricant.
* Laryngoscope, usually with a curved (MacIntosh) blade; a number of sizes are available but for most adult patients a size 3 will suffice (large adults may require a size 4). The bulb and battery of the laryngoscope must be checked regularly.
* Bag-valve apparatus with an oxygen supply and a reservoir bag.
* Catheter mount, to attach the connector to the ventilating device; this may not be required if 15 mm connectors are used.
* Small pillow.
* Suction apparatus, with wide-bore rigid (Yankauer) catheters and smaller flexible catheters.
* Stethoscope.
* Syringe, 10 ml.
* Artery forceps (if using a cuffed endotracheal tube without a one-way valve).
* Bandage.
* Oropharyngeal airway.
* Magill's forceps.
* Introducers (either soft bougies or semi-rigid stylets) may aid intubation.
* Gloves.

PROCEDURE
Endotracheal intubation requires considerable skill and practice and must not be attempted by inexperienced practitioners without supervision. Gloves are worn throughout.

1. Check all the equipment—especially the cuff on the endotracheal tube for uniform filling and to ensure that it is airtight. Lubricate the endotracheal tube. Check the bulb of the laryngoscope. Ensure that all connections are compatible.
2. Whenever possible, endotracheal intubation should be preceded by a period of pre-oxygenation: hyperventilation with at least 85% oxygen for 15 seconds.
3. The patient's head should be placed in the 'sniffing the morning air' position, with the neck slightly flexed and the head extended at the atlanto-occipital joint. Placing a small pillow (about 10 cm thick) under the patient's occiput will help achieve the correct position. This position may not be possible to achieve in patients with a history of trauma and with a suspected injury of the cervical spine. In such a case, an assistant is necessary to provide manual in-line stabilization of the neck.
4. You should complete the intubation within 30 seconds—if this fails, abandon the attempt and re-oxygenate the patient.
5. An experienced assistant can provide cricoid pressure during intubation to prevent aspiration of gastric contents. Pressure is applied anteroposteriorly to the cricoid cartilage, forcing the cricoid ring backwards and occluding the oesophagus against the body of the sixth cervical vertebra. Cricoid pressure should not be used in cases of active vomiting.
6. Hold the laryngoscope in your left hand and open the patient's mouth with your right. Any foreign bodies or secretions should be removed, using suction if necessary.
7. The blade of the laryngoscope is then introduced into the right side of the patient's mouth and slowly passed over the right side of the tongue. By moving the blade of the laryngoscope to the left, the tongue will be pushed over to the left.
8. The blade can now be moved forwards over the root of the tongue towards the epiglottis.
9. If the epiglottis cannot be seen at this stage, it may have been covered by the blade of the

laryngoscope. Withdraw the blade slightly, and the epiglottis should drop down into view.

10. The tip of the blade of the laryngoscope can now be inserted into the vallecula (i.e. above the epiglottis and between it and the base of the tongue). Lift the laryngoscope upwards along the line of the handle of the laryngoscope. The vocal cords can now be seen (Figure 63A). Take care not to lever the blade of the laryngoscope against the patient's teeth.

11. The laryngeal inlet is triangular, with its apex anteriorly and the white/yellowish vocal cords laterally. If visualization of the vocal cords is difficult, an assistant can exert gentle pressure on the thyroid cartilage to bring them into view.

12. Brief suction may be required to clear secretions or vomitus.

13. When the vocal cords are in view, pick up the endotracheal tube with your right hand and introduce the endotracheal tube (Figure 63B) until the cuff is positioned just below the vocal cords. It may be helpful to have an assistant pull the right side of the mouth out of the way.

14. If there is any doubt about the correct position of the endotracheal tube, remove it immediately, re-oxygenate the patient with 100% oxygen, and recommence the procedure.

15. After successful intubation, connect the endotracheal tube (via a catheter mount if used) to the ventilating device (Figure 63C) and ventilate the patient with the highest oxygen concentration available.

16. Correct positioning of the endotracheal tube will be confirmed by:
    • Both sides of the chest rising and falling equally.
    • Equal air entry being heard through a stethoscope held over both axillae, when the bag is squeezed.
    • Equal air entry being heard through a stethoscope held anteriorly over both sides of the chest, when the bag is squeezed.
    • No gurgling sounds being heard through a stethoscope held over the epigastrium, when the bag is squeezed.

17. If the endotracheal tube is inserted too far, it may enter the right main bronchus. In this case,

Figure 63A

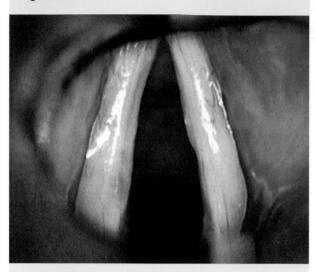

Figure 63B

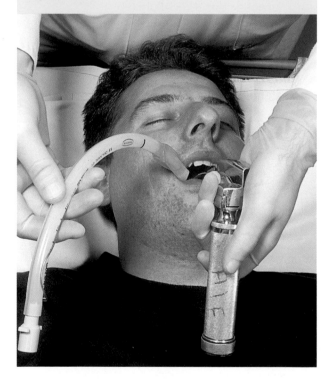

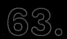

breath sounds will be heard on the right side of the chest but will be decreased or absent on the left. The endotracheal tube should be withdrawn for a few centimetres and ventilation reassessed.

18. When you are certain the endotracheal tube is positioned correctly, inflate the cuff with just enough air to provide a seal (usually 5–10 ml of air), thus stopping any leakage of air. The cuff should be inflated while the patient is being ventilated, so that this can be assessed. When the cuff has been inflated, remove the syringe and, if the inflation tube does not have a one-way valve, clamp the inflation tube with artery forceps. Cricoid pressure can now be released.

19. Ventilate the patient with a high concentration of oxygen.

20. The endotracheal tube can be secured using a length of bandage.

21. An oropharyngeal airway inserted alongside the endotracheal tube will help to maintain its position, and prevent the patient from biting on the tube when consciousness returns.

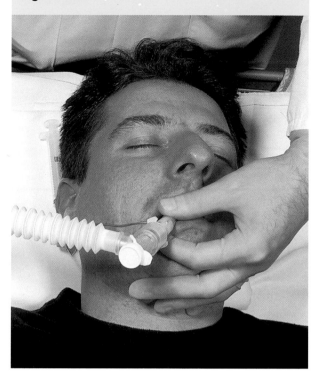

Figure 63C

Needle cricothyroidotomy

USE
- To provide a temporary surgical airway.

EQUIPMENT
- Intravenous cannula; 14 gauge for adults, proportionally smaller for children.
- Syringe, 5 ml.
- Piece of oxygen tubing with a Y-connector attached.
- Oxygen supply.
- Gauze swabs.
- Cleansing solution (e.g. 10% povidone–iodine).
- Sterile towels.
- Sterile gloves.
- Permeable adhesive tape.
- Small pillow.

PROCEDURE
This is an aseptic procedure. Wash your hands, and wear sterile gloves throughout.

1. Attach the syringe to the intravenous cannula.
2. Explain the procedure to the patient. Place the patient in the supine position.
3. If there is no injury to the cervical spine, place a small pillow under the shoulders to extend the neck slightly.
4. Prepare the skin over the neck with cleansing solution, and drape the area with towels.
5. Palpate the cricothyroid membrane between the thyroid cartilage and the cricoid cartilage.
6. Stabilizing the thyroid cartilage with one hand, insert the cannula in the midline through the cricothyroid membrane, directing the cannula 45 degrees caudally (towards the feet), while applying gentle traction to the plunger of the syringe.
7. Free aspiration of air into the syringe indicates that the cannula has entered the lumen of the trachea.
8. Advance the cannula a few more millimetres and withdraw the needle, leaving the cannula in position in the lumen of the trachea.
9. Connect the cannula to the oxygen tubing with the Y-connector attached. Set the oxygen flow meter to a flow rate of 15 litres per minute.
10. Intermittent ventilation is achieved by occluding the open end of the Y-connector with your thumb for one second to allow inspiration, and then removing your thumb for four seconds to allow expiration (Figure 64).

11. Auscultate the chest to ensure that ventilation is adequate.
12. Secure the apparatus in position.
13. There is a risk of progressive retention of carbon dioxide with this procedure and therefore a more efficient airway should be established within about 30 minutes.

Figure 64

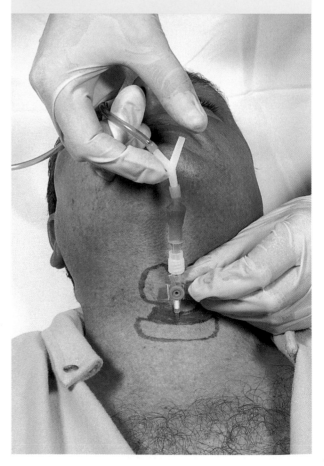

Surgical cricothyroidotomy

USE
- To provide a surgical airway if endotracheal intubation cannot be achieved.

EQUIPMENT
- Appropriately sized (see Procedure 63) cuffed endotracheal or tracheostomy tube with tapes and introducer.
- Ampoule of 1% lignocaine with adrenaline 1:200,000.
- Syringe, 10 ml.
- Sterile needle, 23 gauge.
- Gauze swabs.
- Cleansing solution (e.g. 10% povidone–iodine).
- Sterile towels.
- Scalpel with blade.
- Mosquito forceps.
- Sinus forceps.
- Bag-valve device with catheter mount and oxygen supply.
- Suction.
- Sterile gloves.
- Ribbon for securing the endotracheal or tracheostomy tube.
- Small pillow.

PROCEDURE
This is an aseptic procedure. Wash your hands and wear sterile gloves throughout.
1. Explain the procedure to the patient. Place the patient in the supine position.
2. If there is no injury to the cervical spine, place a small pillow under the shoulders to extend the neck slightly.
3. Prepare the skin over the neck with cleansing solution and drape the area with towels.
4. Palpate the cricothyroid membrane between the thyroid cartilage and the cricoid cartilage.
5. Inject lignocaine (with adrenaline to reduce bleeding) into the area if the patient is conscious and if time permits.
6. Stabilizing the thyroid cartilage with one hand, make a skin incision down to the cricothyroid membrane (Figure 65A).
7. Incise the cricothyroid membrane transversely.
8. Insert the handle of the scalpel into the incision and rotate it through 90 degrees to open the airway.
9. Insert a cuffed endotracheal or tracheostomy tube into the incision, directing the tube distally into the trachea (Figure 65B). Remove the introducer from the tracheostomy tube.
10. Apply suction to the trachea.
11. Connect the bag-valve device.
12. Inflate the cuff and secure the endotracheal or tracheostomy tube using the attached tapes.
13. Ventilate the patient, ensuring that both lungs are being ventilated.
14. Arrange a chest X-ray.

Figure 65A

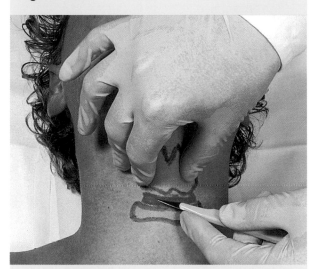

Figure 65B

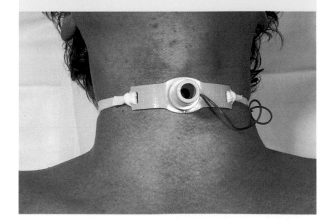

External cardiac compression

USE
- To maintain cardiac output during cardiac arrest.

EQUIPMENT
No special equipment is required for external cardiac compression.

PROCEDURE
1. Confirm the diagnosis of cardiac arrest: there is loss of consciousness and absence of a major (carotid) pulse.
2. Obtain help immediately.
3. Place the patient in the supine position on a firm flat surface.
4. Open the airway by tilting the head and lifting the chin (Procedure 57). Ventilate with two breaths of expired air.
5. Place the heel of your hand over the middle of the lower half of the sternum, that is two finger-breadths above the xiphisternum. Place the heel of your other hand on top of your first hand and interlock your fingers, thus keeping your fingers clear of the chest wall so that pressure is not applied over the ribs (Figure 66).
6. Lean directly over the patient and, keeping your arms straight, press vertically down on the sternum, depressing it by about 4–5 cm. Release the pressure.
7. Continue at a rate of about 80 compressions per minute for an adult. (See Procedure 69 for the appropriate rates in children.)

8. If two people are performing the resuscitation, five compressions should be given for each ventilation (5:1). If you are alone, the ratio is 15 compressions to two ventilations (15:2).
9. Both compressions and ventilations should continue until either the patient regains a cardiac output or the team agrees that further resuscitation is inappropriate.
10. Resuscitation will obviously be stopped briefly during defibrillation.

Figure 66

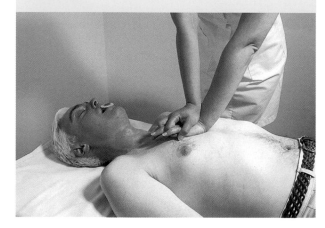

Recording an electrocardiograph

USE
- To record the electrical activity of the heart.

EQUIPMENT
- Electrocardiograph (ECG) machine, with sufficient paper; various ECG machines are available, each with its own instruction manual providing details for recording. A standard ECG consists of 12 standard leads:
  - Three bipolar leads (I, II, III).
  - Three unipolar limb leads (aVr, aVl, aVf).
  - Six unipolar chest leads (V1, V2, V3, V4, V5, V6). Normally, an ECG is recorded at a rate of 25 mm per second. The ECG paper is printed with thin vertical lines 1 mm apart (representing 0.04 seconds) and thick vertical lines 5 mm apart (representing 0.2 seconds).
- Electrode gel.
- Two wrist and two ankle bracelets.
- Chest suckers.
- Tissues.
- Razor.
- Pre-gelled electrode tabs.

PROCEDURE
1. Explain the procedure to the patient, and ask him or her to lie as still as possible during the recording.
2. Make sure the patient is comfortable.
3. Undress the patient to the waist. Shave the wrists and ankles and chest if necessary, where the pre-gelled electrode tabs (or bracelets or chest suckers) are to be applied.
4. If using pre-gelled electrode tabs, apply them to both wrists and both ankles, and apply the chest electrode tabs (Figure 67):
   - To the 4th intercostal space just to the right of the sternum (V1).
   - To the 4th intercostal space just to the left of the sternum (V2).
   - Midway between V2 and V4 (V3).
   - To the 5th intercostal space in the left midclavicular line (V4).
   - To the left anterior axillary line at the same horizontal level as V4 (V5).
   - To the left mid axillary line at the same horizontal level as V4 (V6).

5. If using wrist and ankle bracelets and chest suckers, spread electrode gel at the above positions before attachment.
6. Connect each limb lead and chest lead to the pre-gelled electrode tabs. Ensure that they are connected correctly: the leads will be identified by colour or labels.
7. According to the manufacturer's instructions, switch on the machine and record a trace. Most modern machines will automatically record at least four full complexes of the heart in each of the 12 standard leads.
8. Switch off the machine.
9. Remove all electrode tabs, bracelets, and chest suckers and wipe off any electrode gel with tissues. Make the patient comfortable.
10. Write the patient's name and the date and time on the ECG paper, if these details are not printed automatically on the ECG paper. It may be necessary to label each of the standard leads individually with some older machines.
11. Clean any electrode gel off the bracelets and chest suckers, dispose of the electrode tabs, and leave the equipment clean and tidy.

Figure 67

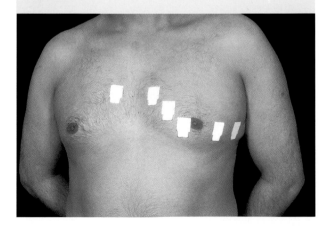

Defibrillation

USE
- To treat ventricular fibrillation (or pulseless ventricular tachycardia) during a cardiac arrest.

EQUIPMENT
- Defibrillator with attached paddles; various defibrillators are available and it is essential that you are familiar with any model you may need to use.
- Pre-gelled pads.

PROCEDURE
1. Confirm cardiac arrest clinically (loss of consciousness and absence of a major pulse) and ventricular fibrillation (or pulseless ventricular tachycardia) on the cardiac monitor.
2. Place one pre-gelled pad below the right clavicle lateral to the upper sternum. Place the other pre-gelled pad in the fifth left intercostal space in the midclavicular line (cardiac apex). Place the pads at least 12.5 cm from any cardiac pacemaker. Remove any glyceryl trinitrate patches worn by the patient, as they are explosive.
3. With the paddles either in position on the defibrillator or on the patient, charge the defibrillator to 200 Joules for an adult (2 Joules per kg for a child).
4. The paddles are placed on top of the pre-gelled pads and firm downwards pressure (equivalent to about 10 kg) is applied (Figures 68A and 68B). Ensure that the synchronizer switch on the defibrillator is switched to the 'off' position.
5. Instruct everyone to stand clear of the patient. Look to check that nobody (including yourself) is touching the patient, either directly or indirectly.
6. Confirm on the cardiac monitor that the patient is still in ventricular fibrillation (or pulseless ventricular tachycardia); if so, press the discharge buttons and defibrillate the patient.
7. Check the pulse and the cardiac monitor.
8. Continue according to the established protocol for the treatment of cardiac arrest.

Figure 68A

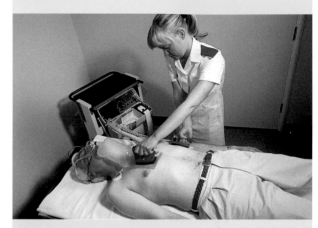

Figure 68B

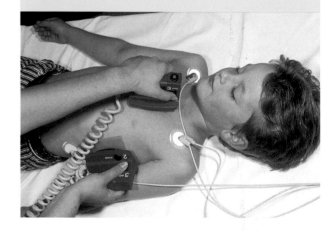

Paediatric emergencies

Some of the emergency techniques described in this book need to be modified for children.

AIRWAY

Open the child's mouth and remove any obvious foreign bodies, avoiding blind finger sweeps as these can push objects further into the airway. Always consider the possibility that the child may have choked on a foreign body (Procedure 62). Otherwise the airway should be opened with a chin lift or a jaw thrust.

CHIN LIFT

Chin lift should not be used if an injury of the cervical spine is suspected. Place one hand on the child's forehead and tilt the head back into a slightly extended position (or a neutral position in a baby). Excessive extension of the neck should be avoided in children and in babies because it may obstruct the airway by compressing the soft cartilaginous structures. Lift the chin upwards with the fingers of your other hand (Figure 69A) but do not press on the soft tissues under the chin, which may push the large tongue back and obstruct the airway.

JAW THRUST

Jaw thrust should be used if an injury of the cervical spine is suspected. Place your index fingers behind the angles of the mandible bilaterally and lift upwards to move the jaw and tongue away from the back of the throat (Figure 69B). The child's mouth can be kept open by gentle pressure on the chin with your thumbs.

INSERTION OF AN OROPHARYNGEAL AIRWAY

A correctly sized oropharyngeal airway should extend from the centre of the mouth to the angle of the jaw when laid on the child's face. In small children, the tongue can be held down using a tongue depressor or the blade of a laryngoscope, and the oropharyngeal airway inserted convex side uppermost ('the right way up') (Figure 69C); this avoids pushing the child's large tongue backwards and thus obstructing the airway. In older children, the oropharyngeal airway should be inserted concave side uppermost, using the same technique as for adults.

ENDOTRACHEAL INTUBATION

A child's anatomical structures are different from those of an adult, so a straight blade is used on the

Figure 69A

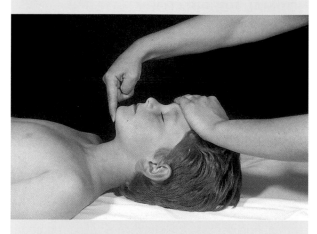

Figure 69B

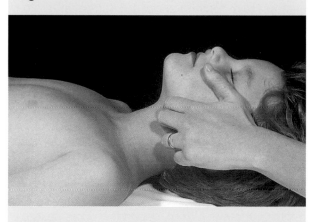

Figure 69C

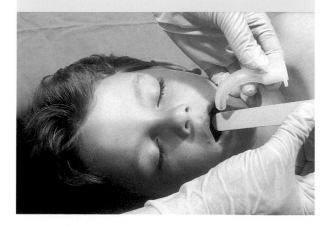

laryngoscope during endotracheal intubation of babies and toddlers. Uncuffed endotracheal tubes are used in pre-pubertal children to avoid oedema at the cricoid ring, which is the narrowest part of the airway in children. In children over 1 year of age, use an endotracheal tube of about the same diameter as the child's little finger or of such a size that it will just fit into the child's nostril.

NORMAL RESPIRATORY RATES
- Less than 1 year, 30–40 breaths per minute.
- 1–5 years, 20–30 breaths per minute.
- 5–12 years, 15–20 breaths per minute.
- Over 12 years, 12–16 breaths per minute.

CIRCULATION
The brachial artery in the medial aspect of the antecubital fossa and the femoral artery in the groin are the easiest arteries to locate in a baby. The carotid artery can be located for older children. If the pulse is absent for five seconds (or is less than 60 beats per minute in newborn babies), cardiac compression should be commenced.

In babies, draw an imaginary line between the nipples, and depress the sternum one finger-breadth below this line. Two fingers are used to depress the sternum to a depth of about 1.5–2.5 cm at a rate of 100 per minute (Figure 69D). Alternatively, cardiac compressions in babies can be performed by encircling your hands around the baby's chest and depressing the correct part of the sternum with your thumbs (Figure 69E).

In small children, the area of depression is one finger-breadth above the xiphisternum, and the heel of one hand is used to depress the sternum by about 2.5–3.5 cm at a rate of 100 per minute (Figure 69F).

In larger children, the area of depression is two finger-breadths above the xiphisternum. The heels of both hands are used to depress the sternum to a depth of about 3–4.5 cm, depending upon the size of the child, again at a rate of 100 per minute.

In babies and children, the ratio of compressions to ventilations should be 5:1, irrespective of the number of assistants.

CARDIAC ARREST
Cardiac arrest in children is most commonly due to hypoxia, which may itself be due to a variety of causes. Most other cardiac arrests in children are secondary to circulatory failure (shock), sometimes due to fluid loss or sepsis. Cardiac arrest due to primary cardiac disease is rare in children.

Figure 69D

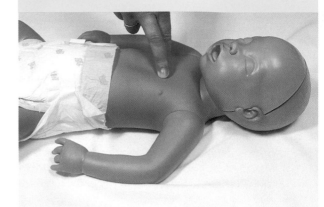

Figure 69E

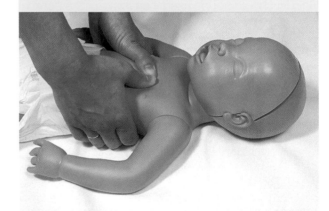

Figure 69F

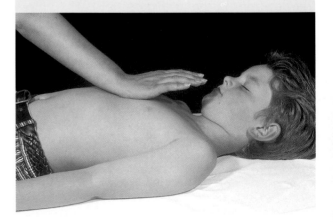

Venous blood sampling

USE
- To obtain a specimen of venous blood for laboratory analysis.

EQUIPMENT
- Syringe, large enough for the volume of blood required.
- Sterile needle, 21 gauge.
- Alcohol-impregnated swabs.
- Tourniquet.
- Bottle(s).
- Laboratory request card(s).
- Patient identity labels.
- Receiver.
- Elastic adhesive wound dressing.
- Sterile gloves.

PROCEDURE
1. Ensure that the correct bottle(s) and laboratory request card(s) are available.
2. Explain the procedure to the patient. Usually the sample of venous blood is taken from one of the prominent veins in the antecubital fossa.
3. Make sure the patient is comfortable, either sitting or lying down, and expose the arm from above the elbow to the hand.
4. Apply the tourniquet above the elbow and request that the fist is opened and closed a few times, to engorge the veins with blood. Gently tapping the vein with your finger often makes the vein more prominent.
5. Wear sterile gloves.
6. Attach the needle to the syringe.
7. Clean the area with an alcohol-impregnated swab (or an alternative cleansing solution if you are taking blood for alcohol levels), and introduce the needle into the vein. You may find it useful to stabilize the vein with your finger or thumb. It is also easier to enter a vein at a site where two veins meet. Apply slight traction to the plunger of the syringe so that you see blood in the syringe when the needle penetrates the wall of the vein (Figure 70).
8. When you have obtained sufficient blood, remove the tourniquet and apply moderate pressure to the puncture site with an alcohol-impregnated swab before removing the needle from the arm. Put the blood into the bottle(s).
9. Continue to apply moderate pressure at the puncture site until bleeding stops, then apply an elastic adhesive wound dressing.
10. Ensure that the bottle(s) are labelled, put them in a receiver, and send them to the laboratory with the laboratory request card(s).

Figure 70

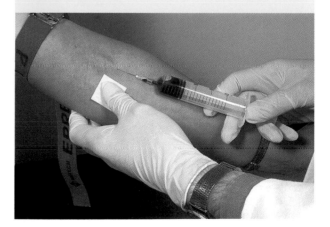

Arterial blood sampling

USE
- To obtain a specimen of arterial blood for analysis of blood gases and acid–base balance.

EQUIPMENT
- Pre-packed heparinized 2 ml syringe with a 21 gauge sterile needle. If this is unavailable, a syringe may be prepared by drawing up 1 ml of heparin (5000 iu/ml) into a 2 ml syringe, expelling any air bubbles and most of the heparin, and leaving only a very small quantity of heparin in the syringe to prevent the blood from clotting.
- Syringe cap.
- Alcohol-impregnated swabs.
- Laboratory request card(s).
- Patient identity labels.
- Receiver.
- Ice (if there may be a delay in examining the specimen).
- Elastic adhesive wound dressing.
- Sterile gloves.

PROCEDURE
Sterile gloves are worn throughout the procedure.
1. Notify the laboratory and ensure the staff are ready to analyse the specimen immediately.
2. Explain the procedure to the patient. Make sure he or she is comfortable lying down. Specimens are usually obtained either from the femoral artery in the groin or from the radial artery in the wrist. Expose the appropriate area.

Femoral method
3. The artery should be palpated in the groin, and the skin swabbed.
4. Place your index and middle fingers on the artery, and ensure its pulsations can be felt in both fingers.
5. In your other hand, hold the needle and syringe perpendicular to the skin. Introduce the needle between your fingers down to its full length.
6. Slowly withdraw the needle while applying slight traction to the plunger of the syringe, until blood begins to enter the syringe. In commercially available kits, it may not be necessary to apply traction to the plunger of the syringe because the pressure of the arterial blood will force up the plunger.

7. In well-oxygenated patients, arterial blood can normally be recognized by its bright red colour (Figure 71A).
8. When the sample has been obtained, withdraw the needle and apply firm pressure over the puncture site for five minutes to prevent the formation of a haematoma.
9. Apply an elastic adhesive wound dressing to the puncture site.
10. Meanwhile, for safety reasons, the needle should be removed from the syringe and replaced by a cap. The syringe should be labelled with a patient identity label and sent to the laboratory immediately with the completed laboratory request card. If there may be any delay in examining the specimen, the syringe should be packed in ice.

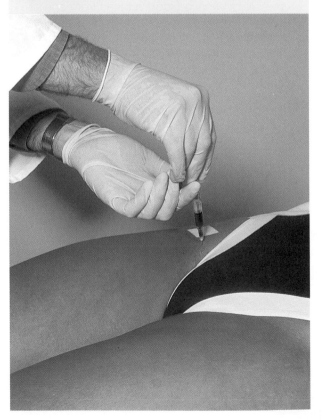

Figure 71A

Radial method

3. Locate the radial artery in the patient's wrist. The patient's wrist may be extended over a roll of bandage to bring the artery into a better position.
4. Palpate the artery and swab the skin.
5. Introduce the needle at an angle of 60 degrees, passing it through the artery.
6. Slowly withdraw the needle while applying slight traction to the plunger of the syringe, until blood begins to enter the syringe.
7. In well-oxygenated patients, arterial blood can normally be recognized by its bright red colour (Figure 71B).
8. When the sample has been obtained, withdraw the needle and apply firm pressure over the puncture site for five minutes to prevent the formation of a haematoma.
9. Apply an elastic adhesive wound dressing to the puncture site.
10. Meanwhile, for safety reasons, the needle should be removed from the syringe and replaced by a cap. The syringe should be labelled with a patient identity label and sent to the laboratory immediately with the completed laboratory request card. If there may be any delay in examining the specimen, the syringe should be packed in ice.

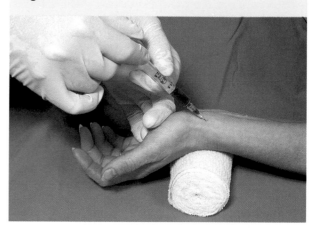

Figure 71B

Intravenous injection

USE
- To give a drug directly into a vein.

EQUIPMENT
- Syringe, large enough for the volume of drug to be given.
- Two sterile needles, 23 gauge.
- Alcohol-impregnated swabs.
- The prescribed drug, together with the correct fluid in which to dissolve it if necessary, and the relevant prescription sheet.
- Tourniquet.
- Elastic adhesive wound dressing.
- Sterile gloves.

PROCEDURE
Sterile gloves are worn throughout the procedure.
1. Explain the procedure to the patient. Ensuring comfort, position the patient lying down, and expose the arm from above the elbow to the hand.
2. Draw up the correct dosage of the drug, dissolving it in fluid if necessary. Change the needle on the syringe and expel any air from the syringe.
3. Ensure, together with an appropriate colleague, that the drug and the dosage are correct and in accordance with the prescription sheet.
4. Apply the tourniquet above the elbow and request that the fist is opened and closed a few times to engorge the veins with blood. Gently tapping the vein with your finger often makes the vein more prominent.
5. Clean the area with an alcohol-impregnated swab and introduce the needle into the vein. You may find it useful to stabilize the vein with your finger or thumb; it is also easier to enter a vein at a site where two veins meet. Apply slight traction to the plunger of the syringe, so that you see blood enter the syringe when the needle penetrates the wall of the vein (Figure 72).
6. Remove the tourniquet and inject the drug, slowly if necessary.
7. Place an alcohol-impregnated swab over the injection site, and remove the needle from the arm.
8. Apply moderate pressure to the puncture site until bleeding stops and then apply an elastic adhesive wound dressing.
9. Ensure that the prescription sheet is signed to show that the drug has been given. Record the time.

Intravenous injections can also be given via an indwelling cannula or an intravenous infusion set (Procedure 73).

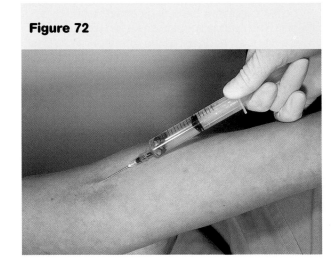

Figure 72

Intravenous cannulation and infusion

USES
- To administer fluids directly into the circulation.
- To provide ready access to the circulation for the administration of drugs.

EQUIPMENT
- Infusion stand.
- Bag or bottle of the prescribed fluid.
- Fluid administration set.
- Intravenous cannula.
- Alcohol-impregnated swabs.
- Tourniquet.
- Permeable adhesive tape.
- Cotton conforming bandage.
- Fluid balance chart.
- Splint.
- Sterile adhesive dressing.
- Elastic adhesive wound dressing.
- Sterile gloves.
- Razor.

PROCEDURE
1. Explain the procedure to the patient. Make sure he or she is comfortable lying down.
2. Ensure that the fluid to be administered is in accordance with the prescription, that the bag is not damaged, and that the fluid is clear and in date.
3. Wash your hands.
4. Remove the protective covers from the bag of fluid and from the fluid administration set.
5. Close the regulator on the fluid administration set.
6. Hang the bag of fluid on the infusion stand. Remove the cover from the plastic spike of the fluid administration set and insert the plastic spike into the connector port of the bag of fluid until it perforates the seal (Figure 73A). Take care to maintain the sterility of the spike as it enters the bag of fluid.
7. Gently squeeze the bag to fill both chambers about one-third full (Figure 73B).
8. Release the regulator to allow fluid to run through the tubing to expel all the air, then turn off the fluid.

Insertion of the intravenous cannula
9. Expose the selected site (usually the non-dominant or uninjured forearm) and shave off any excessive hair.

10. Apply a tourniquet above the elbow and request that the fist is opened and closed a few times to engorge the veins with blood. Gently tapping the vein with your finger often makes the vein more prominent.
11. Wash your hands and wear sterile gloves.
12. Palpate the vein.
13. Clean the skin around the vein and swab the area with an alcohol-impregnated swab.
14. Introduce the intravenous cannula at an angle of 10–15 degrees to the skin, with the bevel of the needle uppermost. Advance the needle until blood flashback is noted (Figure 73C). Continue to advance the needle slightly further to ensure that the cannula has also entered the vein.

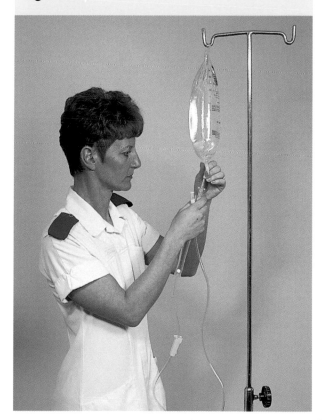

Figure 73A

15. Remove the needle (Figure 73D) and continue to advance the cannula along the vein. Secure the cannula with a sterile adhesive dressing. Blood samples may be taken at this stage by attaching a syringe to the cannula.
16. The tourniquet can now be released and the fluid administration set connected to the cannula.
17. Open the regulator and ensure that there is a free flow of fluid. If the fluid does not flow freely, the cannula can be withdrawn slightly as it may be lying against the wall of the vein.
18. A reliable method of ensuring the cannula is in the vein is to open the regulator fully—this should result in a free flow of fluid. Circumferential pressure well above the site of the cannula will virtually halt the flow of fluid if the cannula is in the vein; if the cannula is not in the vein, the poor rate of flow of fluid will not be changed by this pressure.
19. If the patient complains of pain, the fluid may be running into the tissues. In this case, turn off the regulator and remove the cannula. Apply pressure to the puncture site and apply an elastic adhesive wound dressing. Attempt the procedure at another site.
20. If the fluid is flowing freely, ensure that the cannula is secure. Form a loop with the tubing and secure it to the patient's arm with tape— this reduces the risk of the cannula being dislodged if the tubing is accidentally pulled.
21. Apply the cotton conforming bandage and a splint if required. A splint is almost always used if the cannula has been introduced in the antecubital fossa as movement of the elbow is likely to dislodge the cannula.
22. Record the time that the infusion commenced on a fluid balance chart. Regulate the rate of flow of fluid according to the prescription.

Advice to patients

- Move the limb as carefully as possible to avoid dislodging the cannula.
- Report any discomfort at the site of the cannula.
- Do not alter the rate of flow of fluid.

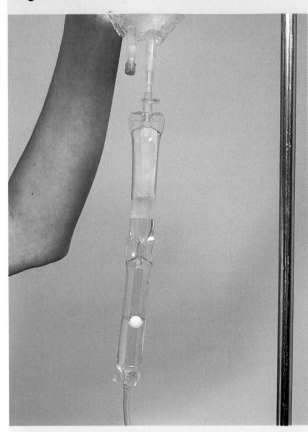

Figure 73B

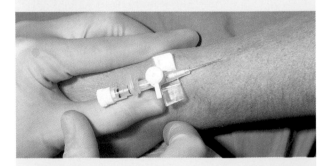

Figure 73C

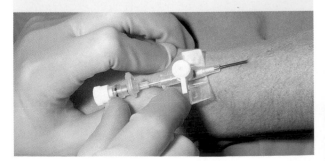

Figure 73D

Cannulation of a central vein

USE
- To gain access to a large vein in order to:
  - Administer fluids or drugs.
  - Measure the central venous pressure.
  - Insert wires for cardiac pacing.

Usually either the internal jugular vein or the subclavian vein is selected. The method described here is the middle approach to the internal jugular vein, using the Seldinger technique.

EQUIPMENT
- Central line pack, including:
  Syringe.
  Large-bore hollow metal needle (select an appropriate length for the approach to be used).
  Flexible guide wire.
  Cannula.
  Dilator.
- Cleansing solution (e.g. 10% povidone–iodine).
- Gauze swabs.
- Sterile towels.
- Ampoule of 1% plain lignocaine, 5 ml.
- Syringe, 5 ml.
- Sterile needle, 23 gauge.
- Syringe, 10 ml.
- Infusion set and relevant fluid (Procedure 73).
- Permeable adhesive tape.
- Suture material and suture set (Procedure 50).
- Antiseptic spray.
- Sterile dressing.
- Sterile gloves.

PROCEDURE
An aseptic technique must be used for this procedure. Wear sterile gloves throughout.
1. The right side of the neck is usually chosen for cannulation of the internal jugular vein, because there is a 'straight line' to the heart, the apical pleura does not rise as high as on the left side, and the thoracic duct is on the left side.
2. If the patient is conscious, explain the procedure. Ensuring comfort, position the patient lying down, with head turned away from the side of the approach. A 15 degrees head-down tilt may help to distend the vein (Figure 74A).
3. Identify the relevant landmarks and cleanse the area with cleansing solution. Towel the area. If possible, identify the carotid pulse at the level of the thyroid cartilage using the tips of the fingers of your left hand. The internal jugular vein runs parallel to, and lateral to, the carotid artery within the carotid sheath, deep to the sternocleidomastoid muscle.
4. If the patient is conscious and time permits, anaesthetize the area with 1% plain lignocaine solution.
5. With the fingers of your left hand still marking the position of the carotid artery, and with the needle attached to the syringe, perform

Figure 74A

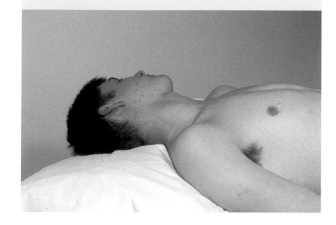

Figure 74B

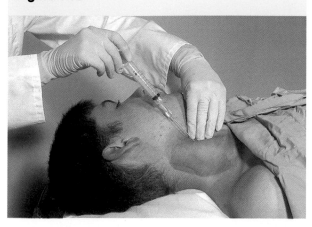

venepuncture 0.5 cm lateral to the artery towards the medial border of the sternocleidomastoid muscle (Figure 74B).

6. Advance the needle at an angle of 45 degrees to the skin, parallel to the sagittal plane.

7. Maintain gentle traction on the plunger of the syringe as the needle is advanced. The vein is usually entered at a depth of 2–4 cm. If arterial blood appears, withdraw the needle and apply pressure for five minutes before making another attempt. If blood is not obtained, continue aspirating while slowly withdrawing the needle.

8. When blood enters the syringe and can be freely aspirated, remove the syringe and occlude the hub of the needle with your thumb to prevent air from entering the vein.

9. Insert the flexible end of the guide wire through the needle and along the vein for about 5–6 cm.

10. Carefully remove the needle, leaving the guide wire in position in the vein.

11. Load the cannula on to the guide wire, ensuring that the distal end of the guide wire protrudes from the cannula.

12. Advance the cannula and guide wire into the vein—hold the distal end of the guide wire to ensure that it does not slip into the vein.

13. Remove the guide wire and attach the syringe to the cannula. Aspirate some blood to confirm that the cannula is in the vein (Figure 74C).

14. A modification of the Seldinger technique is to pass a dilator along the guide wire ahead of the cannula. This facilitates the passage of a very large-bore intravenous cannula, which can be used for rapid infusion.

15. Connect the cannula to an infusion set.

16. Fix the cannula to the skin, using tape and/or sutures.

17. Apply antiseptic spray and a sterile dressing.

18. Arrange a chest X-ray as soon as possible to confirm the correct positioning of the cannula and to exclude the presence of a pneumothorax.

Figure 74C

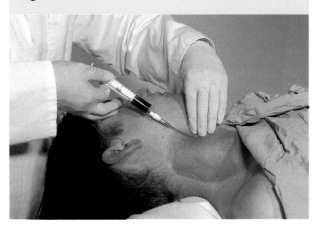

Venous cut-down

USE

- To gain intravenous access, usually in a profoundly shocked patient.

EQUIPMENT

- Sterile intravenous cut-down set, including:
  Scalpel handle.
  Fine toothed forceps.
  Fine non-toothed forceps.
  Two mosquito forceps.
  Small straight pointed scissors.
  Hook.
  Aneurysm needle.
  Small skin retractor.
  Needle holder.
  Towels.
  Gauze swabs.
  Tray.
- Scalpel blades.
- Cleansing solution (e.g. 10% povidone– iodine).
- Skin suture material.
- Absorbable suture material.
- Ampoule of 1% plain lignocaine, 5 ml.
- Syringe, 5 ml.
- Sterile needle, 23 gauge.
- Sterile gloves.
- Equipment for intravenous infusion (Procedure 73).
- Short wide-bore cannula.

PROCEDURE

An aseptic technique must be used for this procedure. Wear sterile gloves throughout.

1. Explain the procedure to the patient. Position the patient lying down, ensuring comfort.
2. Prepare the intravenous fluid for administration (Procedure 73).
3. The usual site for a cut-down is the great saphenous vein anterior to the medial malleolus or the basilic vein in the antecubital fossa, 2–3 cm lateral to the medial epicondyle.
4. Expose the selected area and shave off any excessive hair.
5. Wash your hands and wear sterile gloves.
6. Clean and towel the area.
7. Identify the anatomical landmarks and anaesthetize the area using 1% plain lignocaine solution.
8. Make a shallow transverse incision (about 3 cm in length) over the vein. Blunt dissection with mosquito forceps will identify and expose the vein (Figure 75A).
9. Place two lengths of absorbable suture material under the vein—tie the distal length (Figure 75B) and cut the ends short.
10. Open the vein by making an incision in the vein wall.
11. Introduce the cannula gently into the vein.
12. Secure the cannula in the vein using the proximal length of absorbable suture material

Figure 75A

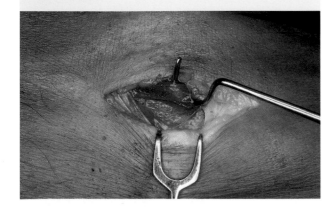

Figure 75B

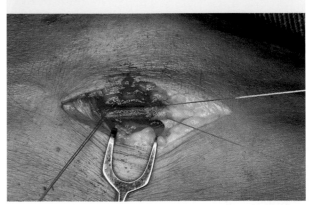

(Figure 75C), the ends of which are then cut short.

13. Connect the fluid administration set to the cannula and open the regulator—the fluid should flow freely into the vein.
14. Close the wound using skin suture material—this can also be used to secure the cannula to the skin.
15. Apply a sterile dressing over the site of the cannula. Form a loop with the tubing and secure it to the patient's arm with tape—this reduces the risk of the cannula being dislodged if the tubing is accidentally pulled. A splint may be used if necessary. A splint is almost always used if the cannula has been introduced in the antecubital fossa as movement of the elbow is likely to dislodge the cannula.
16. Record the time that the infusion commenced on a fluid balance chart. Regulate the rate of flow of fluid according to the prescription.

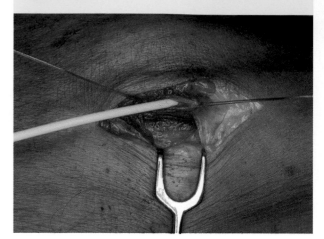

Figure 75C

Advice to patients

- Move the limb as carefully as possible to avoid dislodging the cannula.
- Report any discomfort at the site of the cannula.
- Do not alter the rate of flow of fluid.

Intraosseous infusion

USE
- To obtain vascular access for the administration of fluids, blood or drugs—the technique is used when other methods fail or would cause delay, and is particularly useful in young children.

EQUIPMENT
- Sterile intraosseous infusion needle, 18 gauge, with trocar: at least 2 cm in length.
- Two syringes, 5 ml each.
- Ampoule of 1% plain lignocaine, 5 ml.
- Sterile needle, 23 gauge.
- Syringe, 10 ml.
- Ampoule of normal saline, 10 ml.
- Syringe, 50 ml.
- Prescribed infusion fluid.
- Three-way tap.
- Cleansing solution (e.g. 10% povidone–iodine).
- Gauze swabs.
- Sterile suture set and suture material (Procedure 50).
- Sterile gloves.

PROCEDURE
An aseptic technique must be used for this procedure. Wear sterile gloves throughout.
1. Explain the procedure to the patient. Ensuring comfort, position the patient lying down, and expose the relevant limb.
2. Identify the infusion site—avoid bones which are fractured and limbs with fractures proximal to possible sites. The most usual site is the anterior surface of the tibia, 2 cm below the tibial tuberosity. Other possible sites are the anterolateral surface of the femur, 3 cm above the lateral condyle; or the lateral aspect of the humerus, 3 cm below the surgical neck.
3. Clean the skin with cleansing solution. Local anaesthesia with 1% plain lignocaine will be required if the patient is conscious.
4. Insert the intraosseous needle at 90 degrees to the surface.
5. Advance the intraosseous needle using firm downwards pressure into the bone, with a steady clockwise rotation of the needle until a 'give' is felt as the cortex is penetrated and the marrow cavity entered (Figure 76A). The needle will now stand upright, supported by the bone.
6. Remove the needle trocar stylet by stabilizing the base-plate of the needle cannula and turning the handle anti-clockwise to disengage.
7. Attach a 5 ml syringe and aspirate bone marrow to confirm the correct positioning of the needle (Figure 76B): this specimen can be used for blood tests including cross-matching, but inform the laboratory that it is bone marrow and

Figure 76A

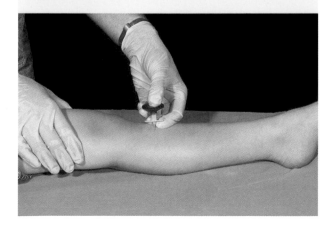

Figure 76B

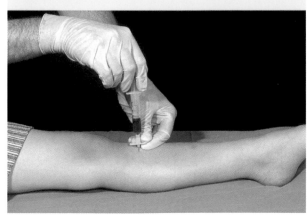

not fresh blood. Correct positioning can also be confirmed by the ease of injection of a test dose of 10 ml of normal saline, without evidence of extravasation.

8. Attach the 50 ml syringe containing the prescribed infusion fluid, and push the fluid into the marrow in boluses. A three-way tap can be used (Figure 76C). Gravity alone is insufficient to force fluid into the marrow.

9. The intraosseous needle can be stabilized in position, using sutures.

10. Intraosseous infusion is not recommended for longer than 24 hours.

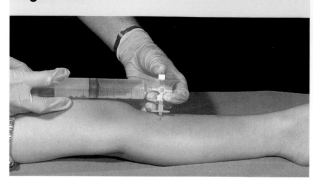

Figure 76C

Dressing for an open wound of the chest

USE
- To provide a temporary dressing for an open ('sucking') wound of the chest. The dressing acts as a one-way valve, allowing air out of a pneumothorax but not allowing air into the pleural space through the wound of the chest. Complete occlusion of an open wound of the chest may result in a tension pneumothorax if there is continued leakage of air from the damaged lung into the pleural space, with no route of escape.

EQUIPMENT
- Sterile dressing pack, including:
  Tray or receiver.
  Gauze.
  Gloves.
  Towels.
  Gallipot.
- Sterile non-adherent, non-porous dressing, of appropriate size.
- Permeable adhesive tape, 2.5 cm wide.
- Scissors.

PROCEDURE
Sterile gloves are worn throughout the procedure.
1. Explain the procedure to the patient.
2. Cover the wound with the sterile non-adherent, non-porous dressing, and fix the dressing securely on three of its four sides with permeable adhesive tape (Figure 77).
3. Observe the patient for signs and symptoms of a tension pneumothorax, including:
   - Severe and increasing dyspnoea.
   - Cyanosis.
   - Distension of the veins of the neck.
   - Deviation of the trachea and mediastinum away from the side of the pneumothorax.
   - Decreased or absent breath sounds on the side of the pneumothorax.
   - Increased percussion note on the side of the pneumothorax.
4. If any of these signs and symptoms develop, remove the dressing and reassess the patient. An urgent needle thoracocentesis may be required (Procedure 78).
5. Prepare for the insertion of a chest drain (Procedure 79).

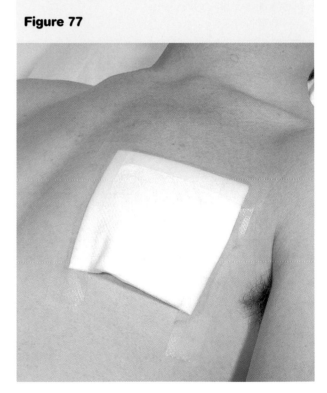

Figure 77

Needle thoracocentesis

USE
- To provide emergency decompression of a tension pneumothorax before the insertion of a chest drain.

EQUIPMENT
- Intravenous cannula, 16 gauge.
- Syringe, 20 ml.
- Ampoule of 1% plain lignocaine, 5 ml.
- Syringe, 5 ml.
- Sterile needle, 21 gauge.
- Gauze swabs.
- Cleansing solution (e.g. 10% povidone–iodine).
- Sterile towels.
- Sterile adhesive dressing.
- Sterile gloves.

PROCEDURE
Sterile gloves are worn throughout the procedure.
1. Explain the procedure to the patient. Place the patient in a comfortable position—sitting upright if possible, having ensured that the spine is not injured.
2. Wash your hands and wear sterile gloves.
3. Identify the site of insertion of the cannula; the second intercostal space in the midclavicular line on the side of the pneumothorax. Remember that the second rib meets the sternum at the angle of Louis.
4. Prepare the skin with cleansing solution, and drape the area with sterile towels.
5. If the patient is conscious and if time permits, inject lignocaine into the intended site of insertion of the cannula.
6. Insert the cannula over the upper border of the third rib in the midclavicular line. The rapid release of air confirms the correct position of the cannula. Air can be aspirated if necessary (Figure 78).
7. Secure the cannula in position.
8. A chest drain should now be inserted (Procedure 79) and its correct position confirmed with a chest X-ray before the cannula is removed.

Figure 78

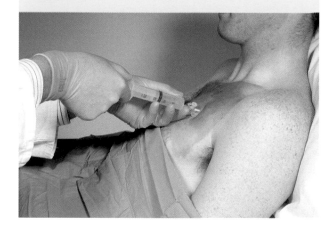

Insertion of a chest drain

USE
- To drain a pneumothorax and/or a haemothorax.

EQUIPMENT
- Sterile thoracic pack, including:
  Scalpel handle.
  Two sponge-holding forceps.
  Artery forceps.
  Toothed forceps.
  Non-toothed forceps.
  Sinus forceps.
  Needle holder.
  Scissors.
  Paper towels.
  Gauze swabs.
  Tray.
- Sterile pleural drainage system, containing a drainage bottle with tubing and connections.
- Cleansing solution (e.g. 10% povidone–iodine).
- Ampoule of 1% plain lignocaine, 10 ml.
- Syringe, 10 ml.
- Sterile needle, 21 gauge.
- Sterile gloves.
- Sterile towels.
- Scalpel blades.
- Suture material.
- Thoracic cannula, of a suitable length and diameter.
- Indelible pen.
- Sterile distilled water, 1 litre.
- Sterile dressing.
- Elastic adhesive tape, 7.5 cm wide.

PROCEDURE
An aseptic technique must be used for this procedure. Wear sterile gloves throughout.
1. Explain the procedure to the patient. Place the patient in a comfortable position—sitting upright if possible, having ensured that the spine is not injured. Undress the patient to the waist.
2. Add sterile water to the drainage bottle. Insert the drainage tube and ensure that it lies below the level of the water. Commercially available bottles have a fill line marked on the side of the bottle.
3. Wash your hands and wear sterile gloves.
4. The usual site for insertion of the cannula is the fifth intercostal space in the mid axillary line.

Ensure that you are draining the correct side! Remember that the second rib meets the sternum at the angle of Louis; count down from this point to the fifth intercostal space. The site of insertion of the cannula can be marked with an indelible pen.
5. Clean the area and drape with sterile towels.
6. Inject lignocaine into the intended site of insertion of the cannula, infiltrating down to the pleura. When the needle pierces the pleura you will feel a 'give' and air can then be aspirated into the syringe.
7. A purse-string suture may be inserted around the intended site of insertion of the cannula. This suture can be tied when the cannula is removed.
8. Make a transverse incision about 3 cm in length just above the upper border of the sixth rib in the mid axillary line, down through the skin and subcutaneous fat (Figure 79A).
9. Sinus forceps can be used to dissect down through the intercostal muscles and through the pleura (Figure 79B). Insert your index finger into the hole to exclude adhesions in the chest.
10. Remove the trocar from the cannula and, using artery forceps to hold the end of the cannula, introduce the cannula into the chest.
11. The cannula must immediately be connected to the drainage system, which may either be attached to the side of the trolley or be allowed to stand on the floor.
12. If there is a pneumothorax, air will bubble through the water in the drainage bottle. If there is a haemothorax, blood will drain from the chest. If the cannula is positioned correctly, the water level in the drainage tube will rise and fall a few centimetres ('swing') when the patient coughs.
13. Suture the wound and anchor the cannula securely with one or two skin sutures, wrapped several times around the cannula (Figure 79C).
14. Apply a sterile dressing at the site of insertion of the cannula (Figure 79D). The cannula can be further secured with elastic adhesive tape.
15. Arrange a chest X-ray immediately, to ensure that the cannula is positioned correctly.

Figure 79A

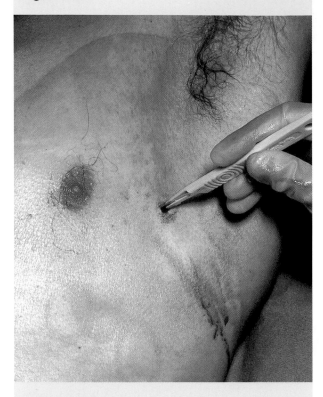

Figure 79B

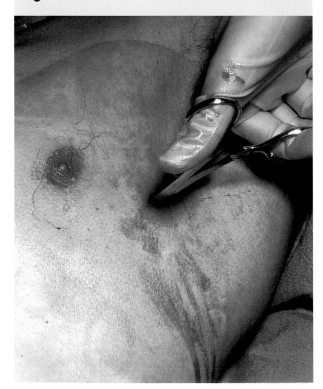

Figure 79C

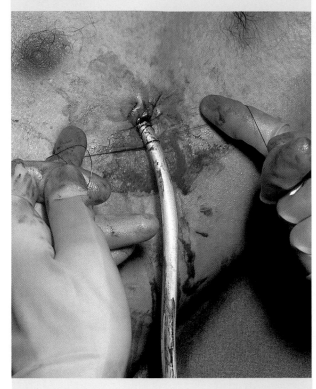

Figure 79D

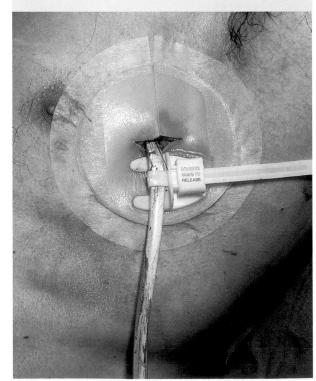

16. Chest drains should not be clamped because this can lead to the development of a tension pneumothorax. However, clamps should be available during transfer of the patient, in case there is a risk of water entering the pleural space. It is essential to ensure that water does not flow into the chest, and the drainage bottle must always be well below the level of the chest (Figure 79E).

Figure 79E

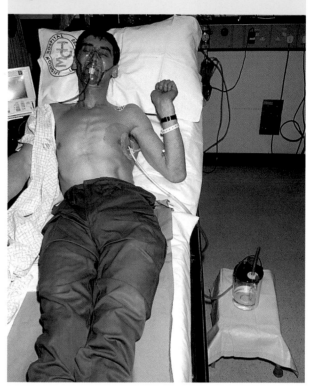

Advice to patients

- Always ensure that the drainage bottle is well below the level of the chest.

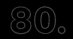

Pericardiocentesis

USE
- To drain fluid (usually blood in the emergency department) from the pericardial sac.

EQUIPMENT
- Intravenous cannula, 16 gauge, 15 cm long, connected to a 20 ml syringe.
- Three-way tap.
- Ampoule of 1% plain lignocaine, 5 ml.
- Syringe, 5 ml.
- Sterile needle, 21 gauge.
- Gauze swabs.
- Cleansing solution (e.g. 10% povidone–iodine).
- Sterile towels.
- Sterile gloves.
- Receiver.
- Cardiac monitor.

PROCEDURE
Sterile gloves are worn throughout the procedure.
1. Explain the procedure to the patient. Place the patient in a comfortable position—sitting upright if possible, having ensured that the spine is not injured. Undress the patient to the waist.
2. Observe the patient's vital signs, and the cardiac monitor, throughout the procedure.
3. Wash your hands and wear sterile gloves.
4. Prepare the skin with cleansing solution, and drape the area with sterile towels.
5. If the patient is conscious and if time permits, inject 1% plain lignocaine into the intended site of insertion of the cannula.
6. Puncture the skin with the cannula 1–2 cm inferior and to the left of the angle between the xiphisternum and the seventh left costal cartilage, at an angle of 45 degrees to the horizontal, aiming for the inferior angle of the left scapula (Figure 80A).
7. Apply gentle traction to the plunger of the syringe as the cannula is advanced towards the inferior angle of the left scapula.
8. Observe the cardiac monitor for any electrocardiographic changes which may indicate that the cannula is irritating the myocardium. If this occurs, withdraw the cannula until the previous baseline tracing reappears.
9. When the cannula enters the pericardial sac, the fluid can be aspirated (Figure 80B). Observe the cardiac monitor continuously during the

procedure, again withdrawing the cannula if necessary.
10. The cannula can be secured in position with a three-way tap attached, allowing further drainage as necessary.

Figure 80A

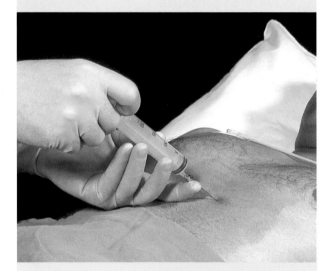

Figure 80B

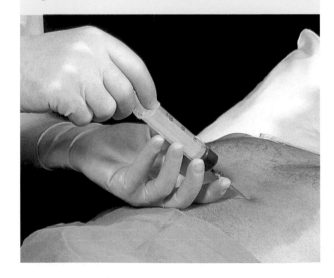

Diagnostic peritoneal lavage

USE
- To detect blood (or other substances) in the peritoneal cavity. This procedure is inappropriate if the patient obviously requires a laparotomy.

EQUIPMENT
- Peritoneal dialysis catheter.
- Equipment for catheterization of the bladder (Procedures 94 and 95).
- Nasogastric tube (Procedure 100).
- Cleansing solution (e.g. 10% povidone–iodine).
- Gauze swabs.
- Sterile towels.
- Ampoule of 1% lignocaine with adrenaline 1:200,000, 5 ml.
- Syringe, 5 ml.
- Sterile needle, 21 gauge.
- Scalpel handle with blades.
- Two peritoneal clips.
- Syringe, 10 ml.
- Warmed sterile normal saline solution, 1 litre, with fluid administration set.
- Sterile suture set and suture material (Procedure 50).
- Sterile dressing.
- Specimen container.
- Sterile gloves.

PROCEDURE
An aseptic technique must be used for this procedure. Wear sterile gloves throughout.
1. Explain the procedure to the patient. Ensuring comfort, position the patient lying down.
2. Empty the patient's bladder with a urinary catheter (Procedures 94 and 95). Decompress the stomach with a nasogastric tube (Procedure 100).
3. Wear sterile gloves.
4. Clean the skin of the lower abdomen with cleansing solution, and drape the area with sterile towels.
5. Identify the site of incision, in the midline and one-third of the distance from the umbilicus to the symphysis pubis. Inject 1% lignocaine with adrenaline down to the peritoneum; this will reduce the incidence of false-positive results because the vasoconstriction it produces will restrict bleeding from the skin and the subcutaneous tissues.

6. Make a vertical midline incision, 3 cm in length, down to the peritoneum. Apply two clips to the peritoneum and lift it away from the underlying structures. Cut the peritoneum between these two clips. Insert the peritoneal dialysis catheter (without the introducer) into the peritoneal cavity, advancing it into the pelvis.
7. Attach a 10 ml syringe to the peritoneal dialysis catheter and aspirate. If more than 5 ml of fresh blood is obtained, the result is positive.
8. If gross blood is not obtained, run warmed sterile normal saline solution (10 ml/kg, up to 1 litre) into the peritoneal cavity through a fluid administration set attached to the peritoneal dialysis catheter, over a few minutes. Leave the saline in the peritoneal cavity for 5–10 minutes. Gentle agitation of the abdomen distributes the saline throughout the peritoneal cavity and increases mixing with blood and other substances in the peritoneal cavity.
9. Lower the bag of normal saline to the floor to allow the saline to drain from the peritoneal cavity—this may take up to 30 minutes (Figure 81).
10. A positive result is indicated by:
    - Blood-stained fluid (more than 100,000 red blood cells/ml).

Figure 81

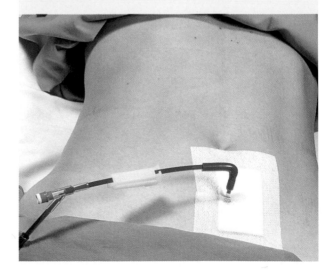

- Faeces, food particles, or bile in the fluid.
- Saline entering the urinary drainage bag, indicating a rupture of the bladder.
- Saline entering a chest drain, indicating a rupture of the diaphragm.

11. When the saline has drained from the peritoneal cavity, the peritoneal dialysis catheter is removed, the wound sutured, and a sterile dressing applied. If the result is positive, the patient should be prepared for urgent laparotomy.

12. If there is any doubt about the result, a specimen of the returned fluid may be sent to the laboratory for analysis.

13. A negative lavage does not eliminate the possibility of a retroperitoneal injury (e.g. injury to the kidney, pancreas, or duodenum) or a tear of the diaphragm.

Local anaesthesia by infiltration

USE
- To provide anaesthesia for minor surgery, e.g. exploring and suturing a laceration.

EQUIPMENT
- Ampoule(s) of 1% lignocaine.
- Syringe.
- Sterile needle, 23 gauge.
- Alcohol-impregnated swabs.
- Sterile gloves.

Usually 1% plain lignocaine is used to provide local anaesthesia in the emergency department. It can be combined with adrenaline (1 in 200,000), which produces vasoconstriction. This is useful in areas such as the face, which tend to bleed excessively. The addition of adrenaline also tends to prolong the anaesthetic effect of lignocaine. Vasoconstriction can result in gangrene if the area is supplied by an end-artery, therefore adrenaline must never be used in the fingers, toes, ears, nose, or penis.

The maximum recommended dosage of lignocaine for an adult is 200 mg (i.e. 20 ml of 1% lignocaine).

PROCEDURE
Sterile gloves are worn throughout the procedure.
1. Explain the procedure to the patient. Ensure the patient is comfortable lying down, and expose the injured area.
2. Wash your hands and wear sterile gloves.
3. Draw up the lignocaine and swab the area to be injected.
4. Inject the lignocaine into the subcutaneous tissues (Figure 82). Ensure that the tip of the needle has not entered a blood vessel by applying gentle traction to the plunger of the syringe; if blood enters the syringe, withdraw the needle slightly and repeat the process.
5. Discomfort is reduced by piercing the skin as seldom as possible, by pushing the needle under the skin edge rather than through the skin surface, and by injecting in different directions through one stab point if possible, by moving the needle under the skin.
6. The area becomes anaesthetized within about five minutes and surgery can then begin.

Figure 82

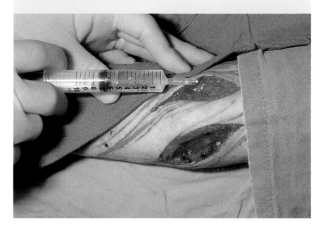

Advice to patients
- Normal sensation may take up to four hours to return.

Bier's block
(intravenous regional anaesthesia)

USE
- To provide anaesthesia of the forearm, wrist, and hand for simple surgical procedures (e.g. reduction of a Colles' fracture); the method can be adapted for use in the lower limb.

EQUIPMENT
- Pneumatic cuff, with attached pressure gauge and equipment for controlling the pressure in the cuff. An ordinary sphygmomanometer cuff is unsafe and must never be used.
- Orthopaedic wool.
- Two syringes, 20 ml.
- Two sterile needles.
- Two ampoules of 0.5% prilocaine (for a 70 kg adult), 20 ml each.
- Tourniquet.
- Alcohol-impregnated swabs.
- Two indwelling needles, 21 gauge.
- Permeable adhesive tape.
- Gauze.
- Sterile gloves.
- Resuscitation drugs and equipment.

PRECAUTIONS
- There are recognized complications of intravenous regional anaesthesia (including convulsions, hypotension, respiratory depression, and cardiac arrhythmias, which could lead to cardiac arrest).
- Recognized complications can be avoided by using the technique described here, and by taking the following precautions:
  - Do not undertake the procedure in patients with a history of epilepsy, cardiac disease, hypertension, sickle-cell disease, known hypersensitivity to local anaesthetic agents, porphyria, vascular disease of the limb, or cellulitis of the limb.
  - Starve the patient for four hours before the procedure to minimize the risk of inhalation of stomach contents.
  - Reassure the patient to ensure co-operation.
  - One doctor is responsible solely for the anaesthesia and the second doctor is responsible for the surgery; both doctors must remain present throughout the procedure.
- This procedure is not advisable for patients under 16 years of age.

PROCEDURE
The patient's written consent must be obtained for this procedure. Sterile gloves are worn.
1. Explain the procedure to the patient.
2. Record the patient's routine observations (temperature, pulse, blood pressure, and respiratory rate). If the patient's systolic blood pressure remains high (above about 180 mm Hg), the procedure may be unsafe and the patient may need to be referred for a general anaesthetic. Weigh the patient to calculate the correct volume of 0.5% prilocaine required.
3. This procedure should be performed in a room where resuscitation equipment and drugs are immediately available. Dress the patient in a gown, and place in a comfortable position lying down.
4. Remove any jewellery from the injured limb and store it with the patient's property.
5. Check the pneumatic cuff to ensure that the pressure can be maintained and that there are no leaks. Check that there is adequate fluid in the control box. Wear sterile gloves.
6. Draw up the required volume of prilocaine according to the weight of the patient.
7. Insert an indwelling needle into a vein in the uninjured arm so that intravenous drugs can be given immediately if necessary. Secure the indwelling needle with permeable adhesive tape.
8. Apply orthopaedic wool around the upper arm (Figure 83A) and wrap the pneumatic cuff over it, ensuring that the cuff is entirely underlaid with orthopaedic wool. Tie the cuff in position so that it cannot become loose or unravel (Figure 83B).
9. Insert an indwelling needle into a vein on the back of the hand of the injured arm, and secure it with permeable adhesive tape.
10. Ask the patient to raise the injured arm for about two minutes, assisted if necessary (Figure 83C); this drains some of the blood from the veins. After about two minutes, inflate the cuff to 250 mm Hg (i.e. well above the patient's systolic blood pressure), and then lower the patient's arm.

11. Record the time at which the cuff was inflated.
12. Slowly inject the prilocaine into the indwelling needle in the injured limb, taking care not to 'blow the vein', which is often very fragile.
13. The arm usually becomes blotchy within a couple of minutes of beginning the injection. Surgery can begin about 10 minutes after injection.
14. One person is responsible for ensuring that the pressure in the cuff remains at 250 mm Hg throughout the procedure; if the cuff were to deflate, a bolus of prilocaine would enter the patient's circulation.
15. Once the surgery has been completed, and at least 30 minutes after the injection of prilocaine, the cuff is gradually deflated over a couple of minutes. Some practitioners tend to deflate the cuff fully and then re-inflate it; this is repeated once or twice, to attempt to avoid a bolus of prilocaine entering the patient's circulation. The cuff should not be inflated for more than about 45 minutes.
16. Remove the cuff, orthopaedic wool, and indwelling needle; the indwelling needle in the uninjured arm is also removed.
17. Record the patient's routine observations.

Figure 83A

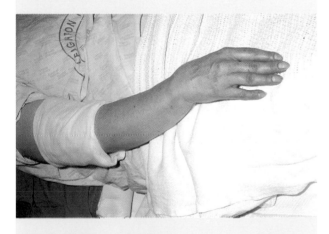

Figure 83B

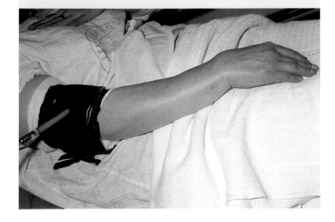

Figure 83C

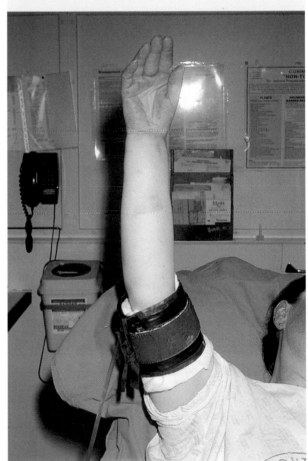

Record the time at which the cuff was deflated.
18. Keep the patient under observation for at least 45 minutes after deflation of the cuff.
19. Ensure that the patient is accompanied by a relative or friend when discharged.

Advice to patients

- Occasionally there may be minor side effects soon after deflation of the cuff, such as a metallic taste in the mouth, tingling in the arm, or ringing in the ears. These effects are only temporary.
- In addition to advice for the surgical procedure, it is important to note that normal sensation will return within about 30 minutes of deflating the cuff.

Haematoma block

USE
- To provide anaesthesia for the reduction of a fracture of the wrist.

The technique involves direct infiltration of local anaesthetic solution in order to block the nerves to the periosteum, bones, and soft tissues. The technique is not effective if the fracture is more than 24 hours old, because by this stage the haematoma will have started to become organized and this will prevent spread of the local anaesthetic solution.

EQUIPMENT
- 1% plain lignocaine, 15 ml.
- Syringe, 20 ml.
- Sterile needle, 23 gauge.
- Alcohol-impregnated swabs.
- Sterile gloves.

PROCEDURE
Sterile gloves are worn throughout the procedure.
1. Explain the procedure to the patient. Ensuring comfort, position the patient lying down, and rest the injured arm on a firm surface.
2. Wear sterile gloves.
3. Draw up the lignocaine.
4. Swab the site for injection.
5. Insert the needle into the haematoma, and confirm its correct position by aspiration of blood into the syringe.
6. Inject the lignocaine slowly into the fracture site (Figure 84).
7. Manipulation of the fracture can begin after about 15 minutes.

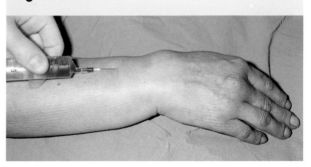

Figure 84

Advice to patients
- Normal sensation will return within about four hours.

Digital nerve block

USE
- To provide anaesthesia of a finger or toe for minor surgery.

EQUIPMENT
- Ampoule of 1% plain lignocaine, 10 ml.
- Syringe, 10 ml.
- Sterile needle, 23 or 25 gauge.
- Alcohol-impregnated swabs.
- Sterile gloves.

PRECAUTIONS
- Never inject lignocaine with adrenaline into a finger or toe, because these have end-arteries and the digit may become gangrenous.
- Always take particular care if the patient is diabetic.

PROCEDURE
Sterile gloves are worn throughout this procedure.
1. Explain the procedure to the patient. Ensuring comfort, position the patient lying down, and expose the injured hand or foot.
2. Wear sterile gloves.
3. Draw up the lignocaine.
4. Swab the site for injection at the base of the dorsum of the injured digit or on the dorsum of the relevant web space.
5. Introduce the needle from the dorsal surface of the digit, skim past the bone, and feel the tip of the needle just under the skin on the ventral aspect of the digit. Withdraw slightly and aspirate to ensure that the needle is not in a blood vessel.
6. Inject about 3 ml (slightly less in children) of 1% plain lignocaine in this position, adjacent to the digital nerve (Figure 85A). The digital nerve is located slightly nearer to the ventral surface than to the dorsal surface but the needle is introduced from the dorsal surface because this is less painful.
7. Repeat the procedure on the other side of the digit (Figure 85B).
8. This procedure will anaesthetize both sides of the digit, all the ventral aspect and the dorsal aspect distal to the base of the nail.
9. If surgery is necessary on the dorsal aspect of the digit proximal to the base of the nail, inject 1.5 ml of 1% plain lignocaine subcutaneously

Figure 85A

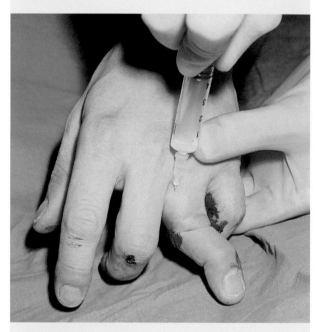

Figure 85B

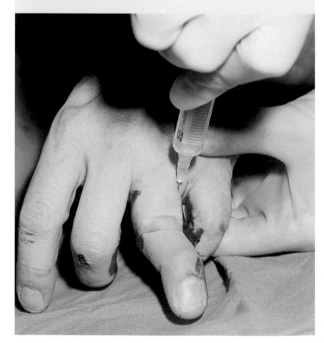

across the dorsum of the base of the digit to block the dorsal nerves as they enter the finger.

10. The digit will be anaesthetized within about five minutes of the injection, and surgery can then begin.

11. The digital nerves in the thumb and in the great toe are slightly more ventral than in the other digits, so inject lignocaine accordingly.

Advice to patients

- Normal sensation will return within about four hours.

Femoral nerve block

USE
- To reduce the pain from a fracture of the shaft of the femur.

EQUIPMENT
- Ampoule of 1% plain lignocaine, 20 ml.
- Syringe, 20 ml.
- Sterile needle, 21 gauge.
- Cleansing solution (e.g. sterile normal saline).
- Gauze swabs.
- Sterile dressing.
- Sterile gloves.

PROCEDURE
Sterile gloves are worn.
1. Explain the procedure to the patient. Ensuring comfort, position the patient lying down, and expose the area of the groin on the injured side.
2. Wash your hands and wear sterile gloves.
3. Draw up the lignocaine.
4. Clean the area of the patient's groin.
5. Palpate the femoral artery. The femoral nerve lies about 2 cm lateral to the femoral artery, just below the inguinal ligament; it divides into a large number of branches just after passing below the inguinal ligament.
6. Insert the needle to a depth of about 3 cm, lateral to the femoral artery.
7. Apply gentle traction to the plunger of the syringe to ensure that the tip of the needle has not entered a blood vessel.
8. Inject 1% plain lignocaine in a fan-shaped manner around the area of the femoral nerve (Figure 86).
9. Apply a sterile dressing.

Figure 86

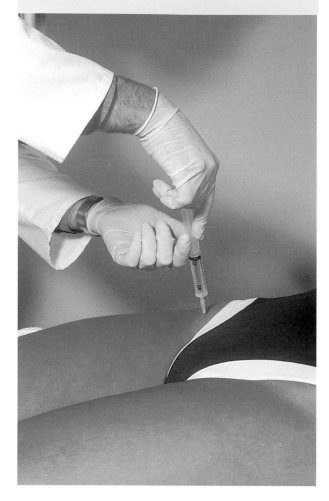

Analgesia with nitrous oxide/oxygen

USE
- To relieve pain and discomfort from a variety of procedures, e.g. removal of clothes from a dislocated or fractured limb, splinting of fractures, reduction of certain fractures or dislocations, application of painful dressings.

Pre-mixed nitrous oxide and oxygen in the proportions of 50:50 in a single cylinder is available commercially; it supplies a constant predictable gas mixture, which ensures adequate oxygenation while providing satisfactory relief of pain.

EQUIPMENT
- Cylinder containing 50% nitrous oxide and 50% oxygen, with a demand-valve and a mask or a disposable mouthpiece attached for self-administration by the patient.
- Trolley for transporting the cylinder.
- Suction apparatus, in case of vomiting.

PRECAUTIONS
Nitrous oxide may have a deleterious effect if used in patients with an air-containing closed space because nitrous oxide diffuses into such a space with a resulting increase in pressure. It should not, therefore, be used if the patient has an actual or suspected pneumothorax because the pneumothorax may enlarge and further compromise respiration. Similarly, nitrous oxide should not be used if the patient has had a head injury, if there is a possibility of a leak of cerebrospinal fluid and a traumatic aerocele.

It is essential that the patient self-administers the gas, so that if consciousness is lost, the patient will drop the mask and so avoid the toxic effects of the nitrous oxide.

PROCEDURE
1. Explain the procedure to the patient, stressing the pain relief which is available if the equipment is used correctly.
2. Make sure the patient is comfortable lying down.
3. Instruct the patient in the self-administration of the gas, through a special demand-valve. The mask should be pressed firmly to the face, covering the mouth and nose and thus forming an airtight seal between the face and the mask (Figure 87A). Alternatively, the patient can place the mouthpiece (Figure 87B) between the lips.

Encourage slow deep breaths. If the apparatus is being used correctly, a hissing sound is heard when the patient breathes in and the gas is released.
4. As maximum relief of pain is achieved after about two minutes, painful procedures should be avoided during this time.
5. Encourage the patient throughout the procedure and supervise the correct use of the equipment. Reassure the patient if lightheadedness or restlessness are experienced, and advise that these symptoms will quickly disappear.
6. Ensure that the mask is thoroughly cleansed and dried or that the mouthpiece is discarded after use.

Figure 87A

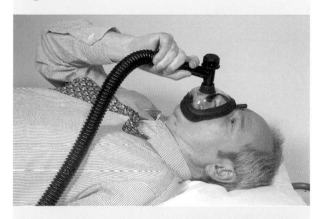

Figure 87B

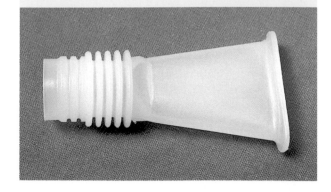

Irrigation of the eye

USES
- To treat chemical burns of the eye. Patients with chemical injuries of the eye should have immediate and copious irrigation of the eye.
- To remove multiple foreign bodies which are not embedded in the cornea.

EQUIPMENT
- Plastic cape.
- Infusion stand.
- Fluid administration set.
- Normal saline, 1 litre.
- Receiver.
- pH testing paper.
- Amethocaine 1% eye drops.
- Fluorescein 2% eye drops.
- Torch with cobalt blue lens.
- Eye pad.
- Permeable adhesive tape.
- Sterile gloves.
- Snellen chart.

PROCEDURE
Good lighting is essential for this procedure. Sterile gloves are worn.
1. Explain the procedure to the patient.
2. Make sure the patient is sitting comfortably in a chair with the head firmly supported in a headrest. Alternatively, position lying down on a trolley.
3. Wear sterile gloves.
4. Check that the bag of normal saline is undamaged, clear, and in date. Attach the bag of normal saline to the fluid administration set, and hang the bag on the infusion stand.
5. Remove the patient's glasses or contact lenses and protect clothes with a plastic cape.
6. If the patient is unable to keep his or her eyes open because of irritation, instil a few drops of amethocaine 1% eye drops into the eye to provide local anaesthesia; this will sting briefly.
7. Request the patient to hold the receiver close to the jaw on the side to be irrigated.
8. Tilt the patient's head slightly towards the side to be irrigated.
9. Hold the patient's eyelid open with one hand and use your other hand to direct a stream of normal saline across the eye towards the receiver (Figure 88A). To enable the patient to become accustomed to the sensation, begin the irrigation on the patient's cheek and gradually move to the eye. Encourage the patient to move the eye around during the irrigation.
10. At the end of the irrigation, pH testing paper can be applied to the cornea to assess the pH when acid or alkaline substances have been in the eye (Figure 88B). Record the result.

Figure 88A

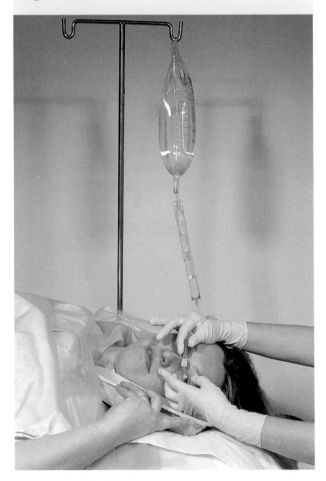

11. At the end of the irrigation, the eye should be thoroughly examined, the visual acuity tested with a Snellen chart, the result recorded, and the cornea stained with fluorescein 2% eye drops to detect or eliminate any corneal damage. When a blue light is shone obliquely across the eye after instillation of fluorescein, an abrasion will be visible as a green fluorescent stain. Any remaining particles must be removed (Procedure 89).
12. If you think the patient requires more expert management, refer to an ophthalmologist immediately.
13. An eye pad may be applied if this is in accordance with local policy, although many experts consider that an eye pad is not required after irrigation of the eye. It should be applied over the closed eye and secured with permeable adhesive tape, applied from the forehead to the cheek. Ensure that the patient is not able to open the eye under the eye pad.

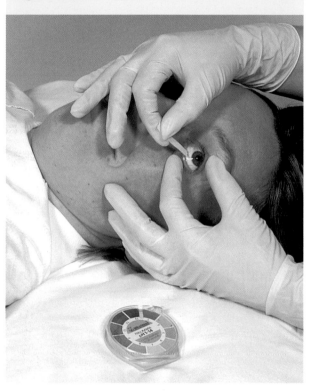

Figure 88B

Advice to patients

- The eye pad must be worn for several hours.
- Do not drive or smoke while wearing the eye pad.
- Wear sunglasses if strong light causes discomfort.
- To use antibiotic eye drops or ointment: wash your hands, pull the lower eyelid down, and apply the eye drops or ointment to the everted lower eyelid.

Removal of a foreign body from the eye

USE
- To remove a foreign body from the eye.

EQUIPMENT
- Snellen chart.
- Cotton buds.
- Sterile needle, 23 gauge.
- Amethocaine 1% eye drops.
- Fluorescein 2% eye drops.
- Torch with cobalt blue lens.
- Sodium chloride 0.9% (normal saline) eye drops.
- Antibiotic eye drops or ointment.
- Eye pad.
- Permeable adhesive tape.
- Magnifying loupe, magnifying spectacles, or slit-lamp microscope.
- Sterile gloves.

PROCEDURE
Good lighting is essential for this procedure. Sterile gloves are worn.
1. Explain the procedure to the patient.
2. Make sure the patient is sitting comfortably in a chair with the head firmly supported in a headrest. Alternatively, position lying down on a trolley.
3. Test and record the patient's visual acuity, using a Snellen chart.
4. Wear sterile gloves.
5. Remove the patient's glasses or contact lenses.
6. Examine the cornea and conjunctiva (including under the upper and lower eyelids) in order to locate any foreign bodies. Use a magnifying loupe, magnifying spectacles, or a slit-lamp microscope. If you think that the patient requires more expert management, refer to an ophthalmologist immediately.
7. To examine under the upper eyelid, ask the patient to look down and gently press a cotton bud along the upper margin of the eyelid. Then ask the patient to open both eyes and evert the upper eyelid by gently pulling the eyelashes downwards, forwards, then upwards (Figure 89A). A foreign body under the eyelid (subtarsal) can then easily be removed.
8. It may be possible to remove the foreign body by irrigation (Procedure 88) or with a cotton bud. If not, the eye should be anaesthetized

using two or three drops of amethocaine 1% eye drops; this will sting briefly.
9. The patient fixes his or her gaze on a stationary object, and the foreign body is removed from the cornea using a sterile needle (Figure 89B). The needle should

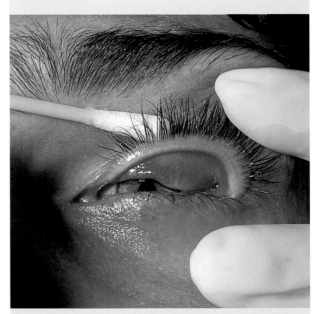

Figure 89A

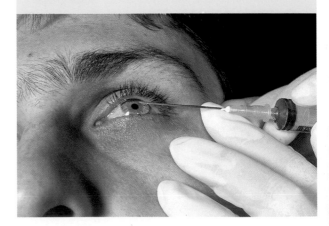

Figure 89B

always be introduced from the side in case the patient suddenly moves forwards, causing a penetrating injury to the eye.

10. A few drops of fluorescein 2% eye drops should be instilled into the eye to detect or eliminate any corneal damage. When a blue light is shone obliquely across the eye after instillation of fluorescein, an abrasion will be visible as a green fluorescent stain.

11. If the foreign body contains iron, a rust ring may remain after removal of the foreign body. This is usually treated with an antibiotic ointment for two days; this softens the rust, which can then be removed with a sterile needle.

12. Rinse the eye with sodium chloride 0.9% eye drops.

13. Antibiotic eye drops or ointment are usually prescribed if the cornea is damaged as a result of an ulcer or an abrasion.

14. An eye pad may be applied if this is in accordance with local policy. It should be applied over the closed eye and secured with permeable adhesive tape, applied from the forehead to the cheek (Figure 89C). Ensure that the patient is not able to open the eye under the eye pad. Wearing an eye pad reduces the irritation of a corneal abrasion.

Figure 89C

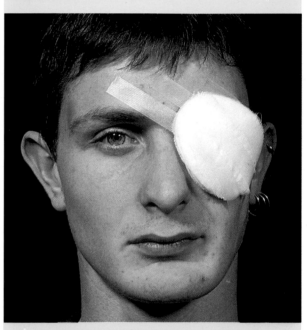

Figure 89D

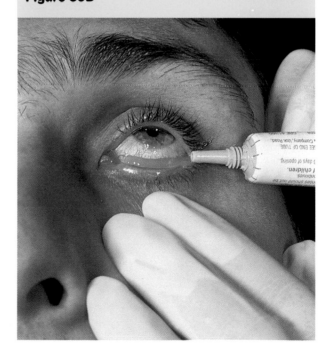

Advice to patients

- The eye pad must be worn for several hours.
- Do not drive or smoke while wearing the eye pad.
- Wear sunglasses if strong light causes discomfort.
- To use antibiotic eye drops or ointment: wash your hands, pull the lower eyelid down, and apply the eye drops or ointment to the everted lower eyelid (Figure 89D).

Removal of a foreign body from the ear

USE
- To remove a foreign body from the ear.

EQUIPMENT
- Auriscope.
- Aural specula; various sizes are available.
- Tilley's nasal dressing forceps.
- Strabismus hook.
- Blunt right-angled probe.
- Sterile gloves.

PROCEDURE
Good lighting is essential for this procedure. Sterile gloves are worn throughout.
1. Explain the procedure to the patient.
2. The patient's head must be held completely still. Make sure the patient is comfortable, either sitting in a chair with a headrest or lying on a trolley. A child may need to be held firmly on an adult's knee and/or in a blanket. Occasionally, sedation or a general anaesthetic may be required.
3. Use the auriscope and aural specula to locate the foreign body and to assess its size, shape, and consistency. Gently pulling the pinna may improve visibility (Figure 90A).
4. It is essential that the foreign body is not pushed further into the ear, and that the tympanic membrane is not damaged.
5. If the practitioner feels that it is safe to do so, the foreign body is removed using forceps and/or a strabismus hook and/or a probe.
6. If the practitioner feels that it is unsafe to attempt to remove the foreign body, the patient must be referred to an ear, nose, and throat surgeon, who can remove it under general anaesthesia and/or with other instruments and/or with suction.
7. It is inadvisable to attempt to syringe a foreign body from the ear in the emergency department.
8. After removal of the foreign body, examine the ear carefully to ensure that no foreign body remains and that the external auditory meatus and the tympanic membrane are not damaged (Figure 90B).

Figure 90A

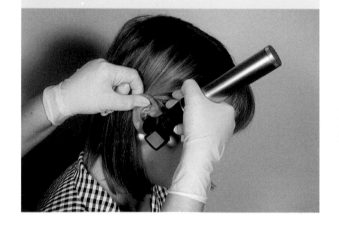

Figure 90B

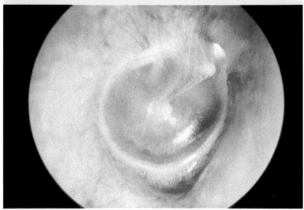

Removal of a foreign body from the nose

USE
* To remove a foreign body from the nose.

EQUIPMENT
* Nasal specula; various sizes are available.
* Tilley's nasal dressing forceps.
* Strabismus hook.
* Blunt right-angled probe.
* Sterile gloves.

PROCEDURE
Good lighting is essential for this procedure.
1. Explain the procedure to the patient.
2. The patient's head must be held completely still. Make sure the patient is comfortable, either sitting in a chair with a headrest or lying on a trolley in a head-up position. A child may need to be held firmly on an adult's knee and/or in a blanket. Occasionally, sedation or a general anaesthetic may be required.
3. Gently insert a suitably sized nasal speculum into the nostril and locate the foreign body. Assess its size, shape, and consistency. A second person may be required to direct a light source up the patient's nostril.
4. It is essential that the foreign body is not pushed further up the nose.
5. Attempt to push out the foreign body by applying pressure on the outer surface of the nose above the foreign body.
6. If this is unsuccessful, occlude the other nostril and ask the patient to blow his or her nose. If the object becomes visible, apply pressure on the outer surface of the nose above the foreign body to prevent it from slipping back into the nose.
7. When using this method with a child, ensure that the child understands exactly what participation is expected. A young child may inhale the foreign body.
8. If these methods have not been successful and the practitioner feels that it is safe to do so, the foreign body can be removed by using Tilley's nasal dressing forceps (Figure 91) and/or a strabismus hook and/or a probe. The nostril should be occluded above the foreign body as the foreign body

is withdrawn to prevent it from slipping back into the nose.
9. If the practitioner feels that it is unsafe to attempt to remove the foreign body, the patient must be referred to an ear, nose, and throat surgeon, who can remove it under general anaesthesia and/or with other instruments and/or with suction.
10. After removal of the foreign body, examine the nose carefully to ensure that no foreign body remains and that no damage has been caused.

Figure 91

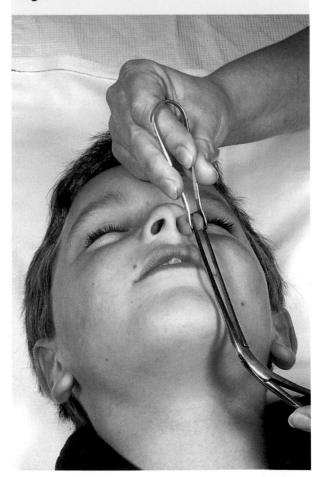

Nasal packing with ribbon gauze

USE
• To stop a nose bleed.

EQUIPMENT
• Bismuth, iodoform, and paraffin paste (BIPP)-impregnated ribbon gauze, 1.5 cm wide and about 60 cm long, or equivalent.
• Plastic cape.
• Receiver.
• Tissues.
• Gallipot.
• Nasal specula; various sizes are available.
• Tilley's nasal dressing forceps.
• Nasal bolster.
• Scissors.
• Sterile gloves.
• Safety glasses.
• Mouthwash.

PROCEDURE
Sterile gloves are worn.
1. Explain the procedure to the patient.
2. Record the patient's blood pressure and pulse rate.
3. Make sure the patient is comfortable on a chair or trolley in a semi-recumbent position with the head well supported but tilted slightly backwards.
4. Protect the patient's clothes with a plastic cape.
5. Ensure that a receiver is available for spitting out blood. Ensure that tissues are available.
6. Wash your hands and wear sterile gloves and safety glasses.
7. Either place the BIPP-impregnated ribbon gauze into the gallipot or snip the package according to the manufacturer's instructions.
8. Dilate the patient's nostril with a nasal speculum.
9. Ask the patient to breathe through the mouth.
10. Using Tilley's nasal dressing forceps, insert the end of the ribbon gauze along the floor of the nose for about 5 cm.
11. Release the forceps and withdraw them. Pick up a loop of ribbon gauze about 5 cm from the nostril. This loop and successive loops are packed on top of each other, filling the nasal cavity both from below upwards and from behind forwards (Figure 92A); this may cause some discomfort to the patient.

12. The packing must be inserted firmly and fairly tightly. At the end of the procedure, the cut end of the gauze should be visible outside the nostril (Figure 92B). Depending upon the site of the bleeding, it may be necessary to pack both nostrils to provide additional pressure to the bleeding point.
13. A nasal bolster is positioned under the nose to prevent the pack from becoming dislodged. The nasal bolster is tied behind the patient's head (Figure 92C).
14. Provide a mouthwash.

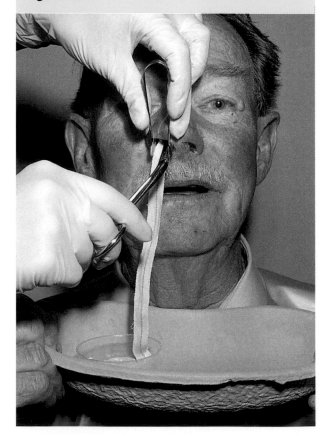

Figure 92A

If this procedure is unsuccessful, the nose can be packed with an expanding foam tampon (Procedure 93) or the patient may require referral to an ear, nose, and throat surgeon, who may cauterize the bleeding point.

Advice to patients

- Leave the pack in position for the instructed length of time (usually 48 hours).
- Avoid hot drinks and hot food for 12 hours as they may encourage further bleeding.
- If bleeding appears through the pack, seek further medical attention.

Figure 92B

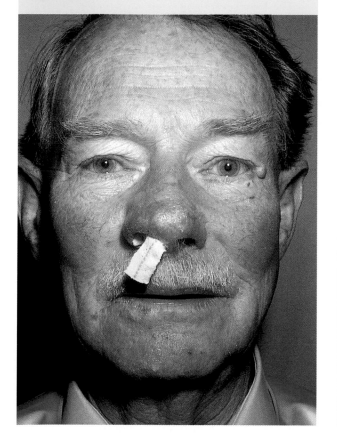

Figure 92C

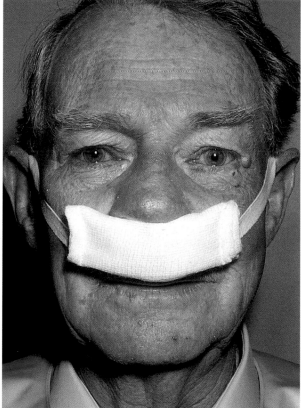

Nasal packing with an expanding foam tampon

USE
- To stop a nose bleed.

EQUIPMENT
- Expanding foam tampon (anterior size).
- Plastic cape.
- Receiver.
- Tissues.
- Tube of antibiotic lubricant.
- Nasal specula; various sizes are available.
- Tilley's nasal dressing forceps.
- Syringe, 10 ml.
- Sachet of sterile normal saline.
- Permeable adhesive tape.
- Nasal bolster.
- Scissors.
- Sterile gloves.
- Safety glasses.
- Mouthwash.

PROCEDURE
Sterile gloves are worn.
1. Explain the procedure to the patient.
2. Record the patient's blood pressure and pulse rate.
3. Make sure the patient is comfortable on a chair or trolley in a semi-recumbent position with the head well supported but tilted slightly backwards.
4. Protect the patient's clothes with a plastic cape.
5. Ensure that a receiver is available for spitting out blood. Ensure that tissues are available.
6. Wash your hands and wear sterile gloves and safety glasses.
7. Coat the rounded edge of the tampon with a thin layer of antibiotic lubricant; the length of the tampon may be trimmed to size.
8. Ask the patient to breathe through the mouth.
9. If necessary, dilate the patient's nostril with a nasal speculum.
10. Grasp the tampon with the forceps or, alternatively, use your thumb and index finger to insert the tampon (Figure 93A) gently but firmly along the floor of the nose until the tip of the tampon remains just outside the nostril. This may cause some discomfort to the patient.

11. The tampon should expand immediately when moistened by blood present in the nostril. If it has not expanded fully within about 30 seconds, gently squirt 5–10 ml of sterile normal saline up the side of the tampon (Figure 93B).
12. Tape the locator string to the cheek with permeable adhesive tape to prevent it from slipping.
13. Depending upon the site of the bleeding, it may be necessary to pack both nostrils to provide additional pressure to the bleeding point.
14. A nasal bolster is positioned under the nose to prevent the tampon from becoming dislodged. The nasal bolster is tied behind the patient's head.
15. Provide a mouthwash.

REMOVAL OF THE EXPANDING FOAM TAMPON
1. The tampon is usually left in place for 48–72 hours.
2. Saturate the tampon by gently squirting approximately 10 ml of sterile normal saline up the nostril.
3. Wait for 10 minutes and then grasp the end of the tampon with forceps and gently withdraw the tampon.

If this procedure is unsuccessful, the bleeding point is likely to be further back in the nose. The patient will require referral to an ear, nose, and throat surgeon, who may insert a longer (posterior size) tampon. Alternatively, the bleeding point may need to be cauterized.

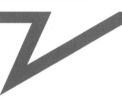

Advice to patients

- Leave the tampon in position for the instructed length of time (usually 48–72 hours).
- Avoid hot drinks and hot food for 12 hours as they may encourage further bleeding.
- If bleeding appears through the tampon, seek further medical attention.

Figure 93A

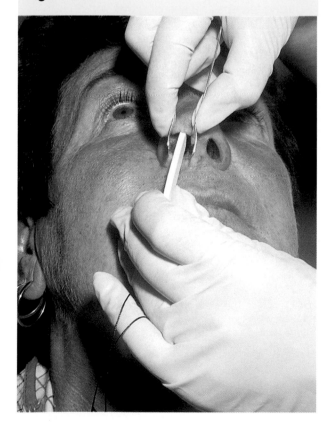

Figure 93B

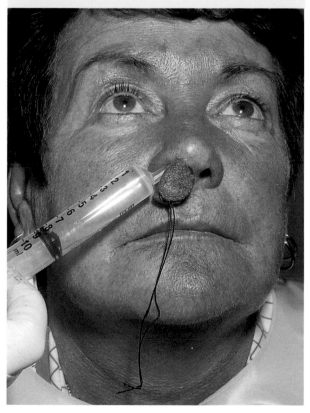

Catheterization of the male bladder

USES
- To relieve retention of urine.
- To relieve incontinence of urine.
- To measure urine output accurately.
- To obtain a specimen of urine.
- After pelvic trauma. Refer the patient to a urologist immediately if the urethra may be damaged, suggested by the presence of blood at the tip of the penis.

EQUIPMENT
- Sterile catheterization pack, including:
  Receiver.
  Gauze swabs.
  Gloves.
  Towels.
  Paper towel with a central hole.
  Sterile non-toothed forceps.
  Gallipot.
- Urinary catheter, of an appropriate size.
- Cleansing solution (e.g. sterile normal saline).
- Tube of sterile 2% lignocaine gel with chlorhexidine and nozzle for insertion, 15 ml.
- Sterile water, sterile syringe, and sterile needle (if a balloon catheter is used).
- Sterile green towels.
- Drainage bag.
- Fluid balance chart.
- Sterile specimen bottles and laboratory request cards.
- Sterile gloves.

PROCEDURE
An aseptic technique must be used for this procedure. Wear sterile gloves throughout.
1. Explain the procedure to the patient.
2. Make sure the patient is comfortable on his back with his legs slightly apart, exposing the penis.
3. Position the sterile green towels (or the sterile paper towel with a central hole) over the penis.
4. Retract the foreskin and clean the glans with gauze swabs soaked in cleansing solution.
5. Place the nozzle on the tube of 2% lignocaine gel and squeeze the gel up the urethra to anaesthetize and lubricate the urethra (Figure 94A).
6. Apply a little lignocaine gel to the tip of the catheter to lubricate it.
7. Place the receiver between the patient's thighs.
8. After a few minutes, gently introduce the catheter into the penis and on into the bladder, using forceps and ensuring that you do not touch the catheter directly (Figure 94B).
9. When the catheter reaches the bladder, urine will flow through it. Collect the urine in the receiver at first until the drainage bag is connected.
10. If the catheter fails to pass easily, do not use force. A different type or size of catheter or an introducer may be required.
11. The volume of sterile water required to fill the balloon of the catheter will be written on the catheter. Draw up this volume of sterile water into a sterile syringe and use it to blow up the balloon.
12. Pull the catheter very gently to ensure that it is retained in the bladder by the balloon.
13. Replace the foreskin.
14. If required, take specimens of urine in sterile specimen bottles, label them, and send them to the laboratory with the completed laboratory request cards.
15. Connect the catheter to the drainage bag.
16. Test the urine and record the volume of urine drained on the fluid balance chart.
17. Ensure that the patient is clean, dry, and comfortable.

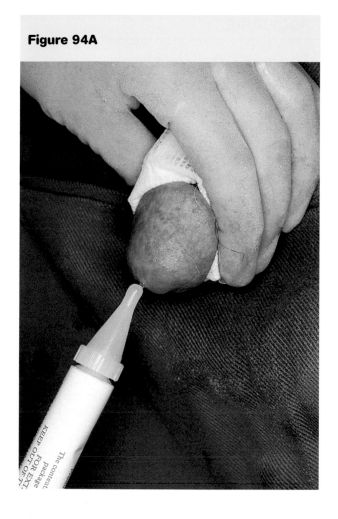

Figure 94A

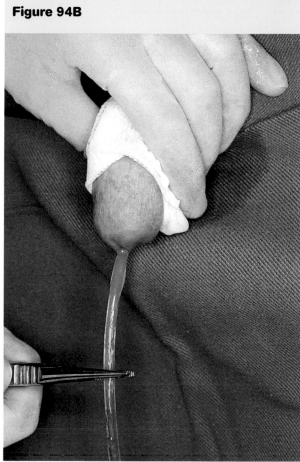

Figure 94B

Catheterization of the female bladder

USES
- To relieve retention of urine.
- To relieve incontinence of urine.
- To measure urine output accurately.
- To obtain a specimen of urine.
- After pelvic trauma.

EQUIPMENT
- Sterile catheterization pack, including:
  Receiver.
  Gauze swabs.
  Gloves.
  Towels.
  Paper towel with a central hole.
  Sterile non-toothed forceps.
  Gallipot.
- Urinary catheter, of an appropriate size.
- Cleansing solution (e.g. sterile normal saline).
- Sterile water, sterile syringe, and sterile needle (if a balloon catheter is used).
- Sterile green towels.
- Drainage bag.
- Fluid balance chart.
- Sterile specimen bottles and laboratory request cards.
- Sterile gloves.

PROCEDURE
An aseptic technique must be used for this procedure. Wear sterile gloves throughout.
1. Explain the procedure to the patient.
2. Make sure the patient is comfortable on her back with her heels together and her knees apart, exposing the vulva.
3. Position the sterile green towels (or the sterile paper towel with a central hole) over the vulva.
4. Separate the labia majora and clean the labia with gauze swabs soaked in cleansing solution. Hold the swabs with forceps if preferred and use each swab only once. Always swab from front to rear to reduce the risk of infection. Swab the labia majora first, then the labia minora, and lastly the central area (Figure 95A).
5. Place the receiver between the patient's thighs.
6. Gently introduce the catheter into the urethra and on into the bladder, using forceps and ensuring that you do not touch the catheter directly (Figure 95B).
7. When the catheter reaches the bladder, urine will flow through it. Collect the urine in the receiver at first until the drainage bag is connected.
8. If the catheter fails to pass easily, do not use force. A different type or size of catheter or an introducer may be required.
9. The volume of sterile water required to fill the balloon of the catheter will be written on the catheter. Draw up this volume of sterile water into a sterile syringe and use it to blow up the balloon.
10. Pull the catheter very gently to ensure that it is retained in the bladder by the balloon.
11. If required, take specimens of urine in sterile specimen bottles, label them, and send them to the laboratory with the completed laboratory request cards.
12. Connect the catheter to the drainage bag.
13. Test the urine and record the volume of urine drained on the fluid balance chart.
14. Ensure that the patient is clean, dry, and comfortable.

Figure 95A

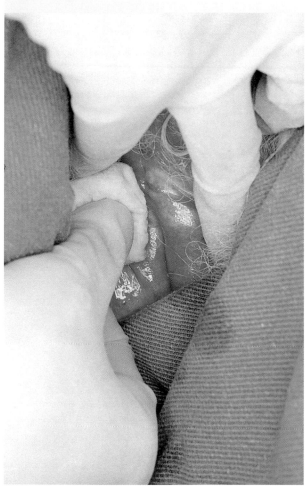

Figure 95B

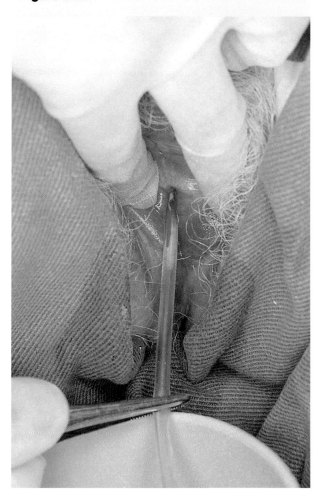

Removal of rings

USE
- To remove a ring from a finger which is swollen or is likely to become swollen.

EQUIPMENT
- Soap and water.
- Length of ribbon, 1 cm wide.
- Ring-cutters.
- Feeler gauges.
- Two pairs of Spencer–Wells forceps.
- Motorized ring-cutters.
- Water-soluble gel.

PROCEDURE
1. Explain the procedure(s) to the patient.
2. Make sure the patient is comfortable, and expose the hand.

Soap and water method
3. Apply cold soapy water to the finger and attempt to remove the ring by twisting it. The patient may find it easier to do this him- or herself.

Ribbon method
3. Slide about 5 cm of ribbon underneath the ring, from the fingertip side to the hand side, using a feeler gauge if necessary.
4. Wind the long end of the ribbon (the fingertip end) tightly around the finger, overlapping each turn, until the knuckle is completely covered (Figure 96A).
5. Grip the short end of the ribbon (the hand end) and gently unwind the ribbon, applying traction to the ribbon in the direction of the fingertip.
6. The ring should slide towards the fingertip (Figure 96B). Steps 3 to 6 can be repeated if necessary.

Ring-cutters method
3. Obtain the patient's written permission to remove the ring by cutting it.
4. Position the patient's hand, palm upwards, on a firm surface. Select the site for cutting the ring carefully to avoid unnecessary damage to it.
5. Slip the foot of the ring-cutters under the ring. Because heat is produced by the action of the blade, it is advisable to place a feeler gauge underneath the ring-cutters to protect the finger.

6. Apply firm pressure to the handles and turn the blade (Figure 96C).
7. When the ring has been cut through (Figure 96D), use Spencer–Wells forceps to separate and gently ease the ring off the finger (Figure 96E).
8. It may be necessary to cut the ring in half.

Motorized ring-cutters method
These are general guidelines: always follow the manufacturer's instructions.
3. Obtain the patient's written permission to remove the ring by cutting it.

Figure 96A

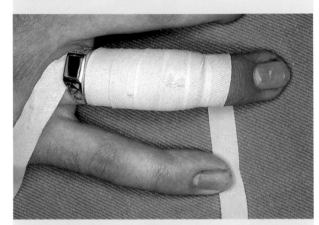

Figure 96B

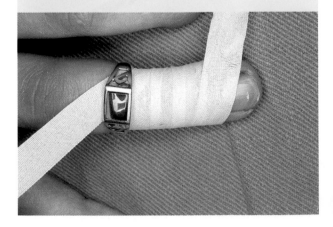

4. Position the patient's hand, palm upwards, on a firm surface. Select the site for cutting the ring carefully, to avoid unnecessary damage to it.
5. Select the appropriate disc for the metal to be cut.
6. Slide the finger guard under the ring, so that the tip of the finger guard extends beyond the ring.
7. Apply water-soluble gel liberally to the section of the ring to be cut; this acts as a cooling agent and dissipates the heat produced during cutting.
8. Place the cutting disc on the ring and switch on the motorized ring-cutters (Figure 96F).
9. While the disc is rotating, gently move it backwards and forwards from one edge of the ring to the other. If the patient complains that the finger is becoming hot, stop cutting, wipe the gel off the ring, and apply more gel before continuing to use the motorized ring-cutters.
10. The speed of the disc suddenly increases when it has passed through the ring.
11. When the ring has been cut through, use Spencer–Wells forceps to separate and gently ease the ring off the finger.
12. It may be necessary to cut the ring in half.

Figure 96C

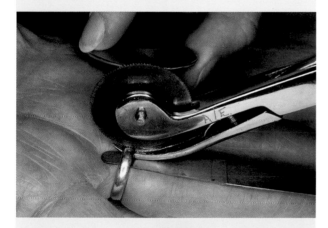

Figure 96D

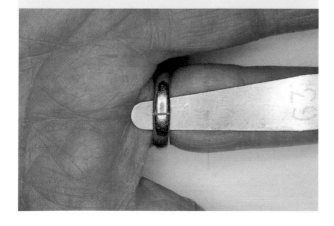

Figure 96E

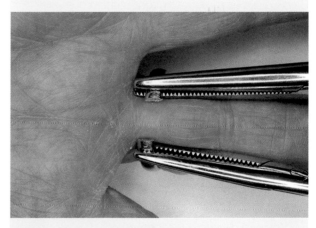

Figure 96F

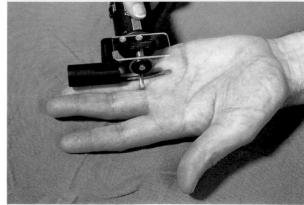

Trephining a nail

USE
* To release blood from under a nail (subungual haematoma).

EQUIPMENT
* Sterile dressing pack, including:
  Tray or receiver.
  Gauze.
  Gloves.
  Towels.
  Gallipot.
* Cleansing solution (e.g. sterile normal saline).
* Spirit lamp.
* Box of matches.
* Paperclip.

PROCEDURE
Sterile gloves are worn throughout the procedure.
1. Explain the procedure to the patient.
2. Make sure the patient is comfortable lying down, with the hand, palm downwards, on a firm surface (Figure 97A).
3. Clean the nail with cleansing solution.
4. Light the spirit lamp.
5. Straighten out the paperclip, hold it in a piece of gauze and heat the tip in the flame until it becomes red hot.
6. Apply the red hot tip of the paperclip to the central point of the subungual haematoma (Figure 97B). It will burn a hole in the nail and blood will escape through the hole (Figure 97C).
7. Gently squeeze the area to express the blood.
8. Apply a dressing (Procedure 44) to soak up any further leakage.

Advice to patients

* Keep the dressing clean and dry.
* Keep the dressing in place for about two days.

Figure 97A

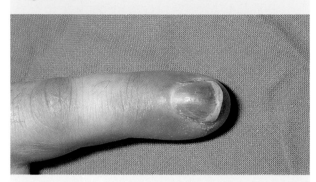

Figure 97B

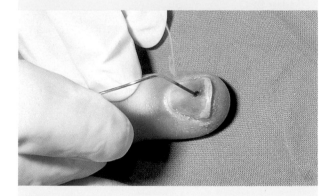

Figure 97C

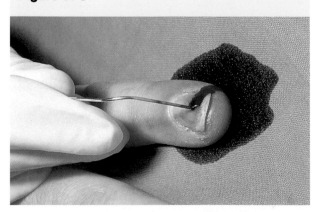

Aspiration of the knee

USE
- To remove fluid from the knee joint.

EQUIPMENT
- Sterile dressing pack (or knee aspiration set), including:
  Tray or receiver.
  Gauze.
  Gloves.
  Towels.
  Gallipot.
- Cleansing solution (e.g. 10% povidone–iodine).
- Ampoule of 1% plain lignocaine, 5 ml.
- Syringe, 5 ml.
- Sterile needle, 25 gauge.
- Sterile gloves.
- Syringe, 20 ml.
- Sterile needle, 19 gauge.
- Sterile specimen bottle and laboratory request card.
- Sterile dry dressing.

PROCEDURE
An aseptic technique must be used for this procedure. Wear sterile gloves throughout.
1. Explain the procedure to the patient. Make sure the patient is comfortable lying down, and expose the leg.
2. Clean the area of the knee with 10% povidone–iodine solution (or with an alternative cleansing solution if the patient is allergic to povidone–iodine solution). Clean a wide area because you will probably want to move your hands from place to place around the knee during the procedure. Position the sterile towels.
3. Inject 1% plain lignocaine solution at the intended site of aspiration, which is usually in the superolateral area of the knee (Figure 98A).
4. Use the 20 ml syringe and the 19 gauge sterile needle to aspirate fluid from the knee joint (Figure 98B).
5. Record the volume and the appearance of the aspirated fluid.
6. Collect a specimen of fluid in the sterile specimen bottle; this should be labelled and sent to the laboratory with the completed laboratory request card.

Figure 98A

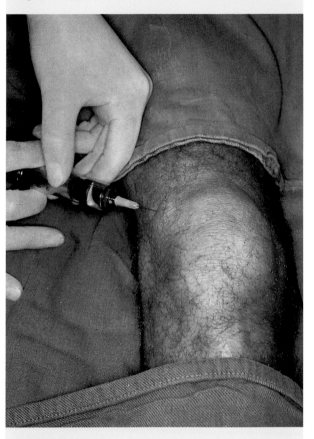

Figure 98B

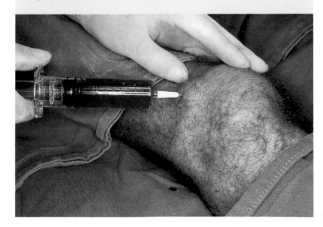

7. Apply a sterile dry dressing to the site of aspiration.
8. Apply an elasticated tubular support (Procedure 14), a crepe bandage (Procedure 16), or a wool and crepe bandage (Procedure 18) to the knee to provide support and to restrict the re-accumulation of fluid.

Advice to patients

- Keep the support bandage clean and dry, and wear it for as long as advised.
- Exercise the ankle and quadriceps musculature by holding the foot at a right angle and tightening the muscle at the front of the thigh; raise the straightened leg for five seconds, then lower it slowly, and rotate the ankle clockwise and anti-clockwise. Repeat these exercises for five minutes every hour, during the day.
- Follow advice regarding elevation of the leg, weightbearing, and mobility.
- If the foot becomes discoloured (other than with delayed bruising), numb, or excessively swollen, or severe pain or tingling develop, seek further medical attention.
- A walking aid may be provided (Procedure 26).

Gastric lavage

USE
- To empty the stomach.

EQUIPMENT
- Trolley, which can be tipped into a head-down position.
- Large bowl, filled with lukewarm water.
- Measuring jug.
- Bucket.
- Gastric tube; various sizes are available.
- Lubricating jelly.
- Funnel, tubing, and connections.
- Blue litmus paper.
- Incontinence sheets.
- Denture pot.
- Sterile specimen bottle and laboratory request card.
- Gown and paper cap for the patient.
- Aprons, gloves, and overshoes for the practitioners.
- Oxygen and suction must be readily available.

PROCEDURE
If the patient is unconscious, an anaesthetist must assist with the passing of the gastric tube, as the gag reflex may be absent and the patient may require endotracheal intubation before gastric lavage, to avoid aspiration of gastric contents.

Two people are required for this procedure.
1. Explain the procedure to the patient. Wear an apron, gloves, and overshoes.
2. Record the patient's temperature, pulse rate, respiratory rate, blood pressure, colour, and conscious level.
3. Dress the patient in a gown and paper cap. Place any dentures in a labelled denture pot. Remove all jewellery and store it with the patient's property.
4. Position the patient on his or her right side on a trolley.
5. Remove any pillows and place an incontinence sheet under the patient's head.
6. Place the bucket on the floor at the head of the trolley.
7. Tip the trolley head-down to minimize the risk of aspiration of gastric contents.
8. Pass the lubricated gastric tube through the patient's mouth smoothly and firmly,

asking the patient to swallow as you do so (Figure 99A).
9. When the gastric tube reaches the stomach, aspirate should come up the tube and into the bucket, indicating that the tube is correctly positioned.
10. Test the aspirate with blue litmus paper; acid from the stomach turns the litmus paper red.
11. If the tube remains empty, check that the patient's colour is satisfactory. If the patient becomes cyanosed, the tube may be in the lungs and must be withdrawn immediately.
12. When you are satisfied that the gastric tube is correctly positioned in the stomach, connect the funnel and the tubing to the gastric tube.
13. Encourage the patient to breathe slowly through the mouth to avoid gagging on the tube.
14. Fill the funnel with 200 ml of lukewarm water, using the measuring jug. Raise the funnel above the level of the patient to allow all the water to drain into the stomach (Figure 99B).
15. Lower the funnel to the ground to allow the water and gastric contents to flow back into the funnel. Empty the contents into the bucket, ensuring that at least 200 ml is returned (Figure 99C).

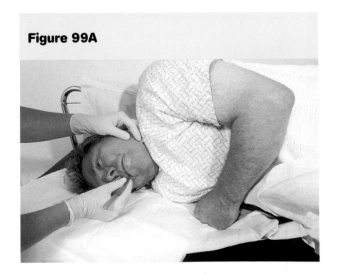

Figure 99A

16. Continue until the water coming back is clear, using 500 ml of water each time. Ensure that the volume being returned is equal to or greater than the volume being introduced.
17. It may be necessary to apply suction to the patient's mouth to clear secretions as the procedure continues.
18. Disconnect the funnel and tubing from the gastric tube. At this stage, activated charcoal (see below) can be poured down the tube if required.
19. Gently but firmly remove the gastric tube.
20. Make sure the patient is comfortable, and again record temperature, pulse rate, respiratory rate, blood pressure, colour, and conscious level.
21. Record the contents of the gastric aspirate and send a sample in a labelled specimen bottle for laboratory analysis, if required. It is preferable to send a sample which was obtained at an early stage in the procedure.

Figure 99B

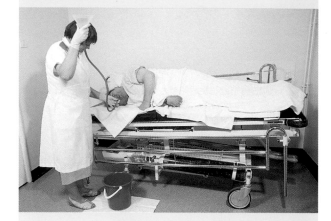

Figure 99C

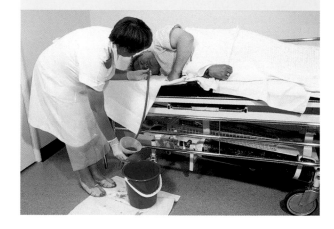

ACTIVATED CHARCOAL GRANULES

Activated charcoal granules are used as an emergency treatment for acute poisoning with certain substances. Given orally, activated charcoal binds with many poisons in the stomach, thereby reducing their absorption. Repeated doses of activated charcoal enhance the elimination of certain drugs after they have been absorbed. Charcoal granules may be indicated following gastric lavage; the suspension may be poured directly down the gastric tube, using the applicator provided in the pack. Alternatively, activated charcoal granules can be mixed with water and swallowed as a suspension. Consult a poisons centre to ascertain specific indications and dosages.

IPECACUANHA

Syrup of ipecacuanha is used to induce vomiting following poisoning. It must be avoided if the poison is corrosive or a petroleum product, because of the risk of aspiration. It must also be avoided if the poison is liable to cause rapid onset of coma or convulsions. It is indicated only if the patient is fully conscious. Syrup of ipecacuanha is taken orally, followed by a drink of water or fruit juice. It induces vomiting within about 20 minutes. It can be repeated if necessary. Consult a poisons centre to ascertain specific indications and dosages.

Passing a nasogastric (Ryle's) tube

USES
- To decompress the stomach, to alleviate vomiting, and to protect the airway.
- To obtain a sample of gastric contents for measurement and analysis.

If the patient is suspected to have a fracture of the base of the skull, this procedure should not be performed as there is a risk of penetrating the brain.

EQUIPMENT
- Nasogastric tube; there is a variety of diameters, each marked at centimetre intervals.
- Jug of cold water.
- Tube of water-soluble jelly.
- Cup of water.
- Bladder-tip syringe, 50 ml.
- Blue litmus paper.
- Elastic adhesive tape, 2.5 cm wide.
- Drainage bag.
- Spigot.
- Safety pin.
- Sterile gloves.

PROCEDURE
If the patient is unconscious, an anaesthetist may need to assist with the passing of the nasogastric tube, as the gag reflex may be absent and the patient may require endotracheal intubation before the nasogastric tube is passed, to avoid aspiration of gastric contents.

Sterile gloves are worn throughout the procedure.

1. If the patient is conscious, explain the procedure. It is important to gain full co-operation by encouraging the patient to relax, to breathe deeply, and to swallow when instructed to do so. Wear sterile gloves.
2. Estimate the length of nasogastric tube required to reach the stomach by measuring from the patient's earlobe to the bridge of the nose and from the bridge of the nose down to the xiphisternum. Note the relevant centimetre mark on the nasogastric tube.
3. The nasogastric tube can be placed in a jug of cold water to stiffen and lubricate it, so that it is less likely to curl up. Alternatively, a thin layer of water-soluble jelly can be smeared along the nasogastric tube.
4. If convenient, sit the patient upright.
5. Introduce the nasogastric tube through one nostril, directing it almost horizontally towards the back of the nose (Figure 100A).
6. Ask the patient to swallow when the nasogastric tube is felt at the back of the throat. As the patient swallows, advance the nasogastric tube slowly but firmly. Giving the patient a sip of water at this stage may make the swallowing easier. Take care not to advance the nasogastric tube too quickly, because it may curl up in the pharynx and cause gagging. If the patient gags or chokes or experiences respiratory distress, withdraw the nasogastric tube immediately.
7. When the relevant centimetre mark on the nasogastric tube is at the entrance of the nostril, gastric contents may be visible in the tube. If not, a bladder-tip syringe is attached to the end of the nasogastric tube and a small amount of gastric contents aspirated (Figure 100B). Confirm that this specimen is acidic by testing it with blue litmus paper, which should turn red.
8. Tape the nasogastric tube to the patient's nose with elastic adhesive tape.
9. Attach the end of the nasogastric tube to a drainage bag (Figure 100C). Alternatively, put a spigot into the end of the nasogastric tube.
10. Attach the drainage bag to the patient's clothing with a safety pin.

Figure 100A

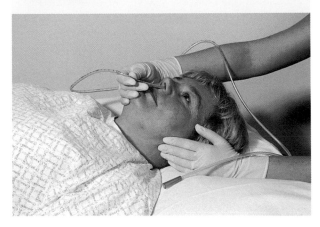

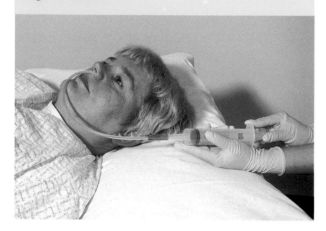

Figure 100B

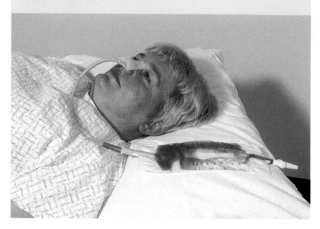

Figure 100C

Index

Index

Index

Index